WORKING WITH PARENTS IN CHILD PSYCHOTHERAPY

Elisa Bronfman
Johanna D. Sagarin

THE GUILFORD PRESS
New York London

Published by The Guilford Press
A Division of Guilford Publications, Inc.
www.guilford.com

Printed in the United States of America

This book is printed on acid-free paper.

Last digit is print number: 9 8 7 6 5 4 3 2 1

Library of Congress Cataloging-in-Publication Data is available from the publisher.

ISBN 978-1-4625-5447-8 (paperback)
ISBN 978-1-4625-5578-9 (cloth)

About the Authors

Elisa Bronfman, PhD, is a senior staff psychologist at Boston Children's Hospital, where she specializes in supporting children, teens, and families coping with medical illness. In her 25 years at the hospital, she has provided training, supervision, and individual and family psychotherapy, as well as conducted numerous patient and caregiver groups targeting a range of child issues, including coping with medical illness, managing behavioral issues, building executive functioning, coping with anxiety and emotional dysregulation, and transitioning to adult care. Dr. Bronfman is also Assistant Professor in the Department of Psychiatry at Harvard Medical School; first author of the Atypical Maternal Behavior Instrument for Assessment and Classification (AMBIANCE), a research tool used to assess parent–infant attachment, on which she provides training nationally and internationally; and coauthor of publications appearing in both peer-reviewed and non-peer-reviewed journals and books on a range of topics.

Johanna D. Sagarin, PhD, is Assistant Professor in the Department of Psychology at Assumption University and a psychologist in private practice. After working at Boston Children's Hospital, Dr. Sagarin was Vice President of Children's Friend, in Worcester, Massachusetts, where she directed their community mental health clinic specializing in youth and families for close to two decades. In this setting, she helped develop specialized programs in grief and in working with LGBTQIA+ youth and their families. She has supervised and consulted with many clinicians; been active in teaching at the university level for many years; and given numerous trainings and workshops for both the professional and lay communities.

Acknowledgments

This book started with a simple suggestion from a mentor: "Why don't you write a book?" Thank you, Gerry Koocher! On a walk the Saturday afterward in Lincoln Conservation Lands, it progressed to "Why don't we write it together?" We are deeply indebted to Gerry for this call to action, which he followed with quick, sensible, and knowledgeable feedback on how to make this book a reality. Part of his tutelage included how to reach out to publishers and editors, which helped us to find Kitty Moore of The Guilford Press, whose early suggestions went well beyond typical editing to inspire and drive us to make this book as detailed, structured, and clear as it is. Katherine Sommer helped us bring the book to its final form. We appreciate the assistance of Manoah Finston on early chapter drafts and Anna Bristow, who worked on the entire manuscript. We are grateful to each other, since it took the two of us to drive it to the finish line.

We have learned much along the way, both from the humbling experience of parenting our own children and from the many wonderful parents, children, and teens we have had the good fortune to work with in our combined 50-plus years of practice. We are thankful for our clients, who have trusted us with their stories and have utilized our suggestions, which have become the backbone of this book. We hope that by sharing our knowledge and experience with other clinicians we will empower professionals to help many families going forward.

Elisa's Acknowledgments: I would like to thank my family for being on this incredible journey with me. Though my parents, Larry and Judith, are not living, I continue to benefit from their many parenting gifts. My sister, Nina, has been a sounding board for me throughout my life, including helping me decipher ways to improve my own parenting. I am also grateful to my daughter, Amelia, who, with unending charm, provided so many life lessons.

There are so many people who helped me figure out parenting both in my role as a psychologist expert and as a parent. I am indebted to my colleagues at Boston Children's Hospital (Annie Banks, Gail Windmueller, and Kate Ullman-Shade) and my attachment research partners (Karlen Lyons-Ruth and Sheri Madigan) for more than 20 years of collaboration. Theresa Ostler provided valuable feedback at the start. Other friends, both mental health experts and fellow journeymen, who tirelessly examined the art and science of parenting with me include Mariko Sakurai, Kimbell DiCero, Diane O'Donoghue, Adam Blumenthal, Lynn Feasley, Marta Siberio, Heather Kelly, Linda Murphy, and Jim and Nancy Boros.

Johanna's Acknowledgments: I count myself very lucky for the parenting I experienced growing up. My parents, Pat and Fred, provided the secure base that allowed me to venture forth in my life. My wonderful co-parent and life partner, Phil, has been nothing but supportive as my evenings and weekends focused on writing rather than on anything else we might have been doing together. I have shared ideas and support with my brothers, Brad and Eric, about life and parenting (and our own parents). Of course, my children, Maya and Jonah, now young adults, have offered some challenges and immeasurable joy. Thank you to all of you.

My contributions to this book would not have been possible without the years of conversations with colleagues, supervisors, and supervisees. I cannot name all of you, but please know that I appreciate the impact you have had on my life and my work. I am grateful to all of my talented Children's Friend colleagues, including Veronica Listerud, Jan Girard, and Karen Ludington, as well as the phenomenal clinical and support staff. I also want to mention Jennifer Denaro, Nevila Weagle, and Nicholas Rotolo, some of the most gifted clinicians I know, as well as Melissa Johnson and Chris Cooper, who, aside from engaging in deep and challenging conversations about our field, have been so supportive throughout the process of writing this book.

Contents

Purchasers of this book can download and print enlarged versions of the worksheets at *www.guilford.com/bronfman-forms* for personal use or use with clients (see copyright page for details).

Introduction

An Integrative Approach to Parent Guidance

A couple, Steven and Cassie, came in for parent guidance. Their child, Erika (9 years old), had been in psychotherapy, but it did not yield the desired results. She was having difficulty engaging with the therapist and was not following through on therapeutic recommendations. Erika was one of five children and, while several of the children had behavioral challenges, Erika was the one identified as having the most significant difficulties. She had trouble with affect management, leading to multiple daily outbursts; when she felt slighted, she became angry and targeted other family members and their property. When her parents brought her for individual psychotherapy, they expected she would learn to control her emotions and behaviors, which would improve family life for everyone in the household. However, this individual therapy did not pan out as they hoped.

Erika's individual therapist recognized that there were barriers to making progress using stand-alone individual therapy. Erika enjoyed speaking to the therapist about her interests and school friendships. When the topic of her behavior at home was raised, she disengaged. Her parents, though well intentioned, were unsure about how to manage her outbursts, vacillating between punishments and "giving in" to keep the family peace. Erika did not share her family's perspective on her difficulties and, therefore, was not as engaged in solutions toward change. She felt justified in her behavior. Erika's therapist believed she would benefit from a combination of individual therapy and parent guidance.

The Need for Parent Guidance

In situations such as Erika's, the child is often the person in whom we are looking for behavior, mood, or functional change. Even so, the best way to achieve change is sometimes through work with the caregivers. If the parents are more skillful in interacting with their child, the child will function better. The evidence is clear: Different "brands" of parent training have been found to be very effective. There is convincing support for the idea that working with parents helps improve child mental health by assisting parents in understanding their children, in effectively using rewards and punishments, in enhancing family relationships, and in establishing healthy routines. This is borne out by research in models that include parent training as an integral element of the program (McNeil & Hembree-Kigin, 2010; Blaustein & Kinniburgh, 2010; Mabe et al., 2001; Lieneman et al., 2017).

When to Recommend Parent Guidance

Parent guidance can be helpful either when the child is not likely to implement changes on their own because they are very young, developmentally immature, unwilling, or unavailable, or when improving the parents' skills in responding to their child's difficult behavior will be helpful for both parent and child, for example, when parents need help managing their own emotions and behaviors in response to their children. Often helping the parent improve the relationship with their child is either an explicit goal or will help them to achieve other goals. Such an intervention can be done either as stand-alone parent guidance or as an adjunct to ongoing child psychotherapy.

Stand-Alone Parent Guidance

Stand-alone parent guidance occurs when the therapy aims to change something for the child but is delivered to the caregivers without accompanying child therapy. There are many reasons that this may be a good choice:

- Parents seek it out. When caregivers are aware that their behavior has an impact on their child's functioning, they may request direct intervention to gain parenting skills.
- The child is unable or unwilling to engage in their own therapy. When the child is not an avenue for the intervention, often the parent can make changes that will help at home.
- The parent is more capable than the child to solve the problems. Because parents are often very motivated to promote family changes, they often implement suggestions more consistently than child patients do. Their cognitive development, as adults, may also provide a wider access to a range of intervention choices that would not be available to children.
- Child therapy has not yielded positive results. If a trial of child therapy fails to demonstrate expectable progress, parent guidance is another intervention to suggest.

Parent Guidance as an Adjunct to Ongoing Child Therapy

Sometimes child therapy and parent guidance are more effective when delivered at the same time. In some situations, it makes sense for the child's therapist to provide the parent guidance, while sometimes a referral to a different therapist may be warranted. When the same therapist provides the parent guidance and the individual child therapy, you can either have regular, separate meetings with the parent or meet with the parent at the start or the end of the child's session. This arrangement is different from having ongoing regular meetings with the parent and the child together, as in family therapy. Adjunctive parent guidance is effective when:

- There is too much conflict in the parent–child relationship for the individual child therapy to be effective. Under these circumstances, feedback, including perspective taking, for both parent and child may assist in shifting the child's treatment.
- The parent's response to the child's feelings and behavior is exacerbating the problem. Having a little time with the parent may allow you to provide a window into the child's experience in a way that promotes a parental change in strategy and emotions.
- When the child would like assistance in sharing therapy topics with the parent and the parent would benefit from coaching on how to behave in that discussion.

Supporting the Child's Treatment through Parent Guidance

An important role of parent guidance, once you have chosen it, is to enhance the efficacy of interventions that the child is receiving in their own individual psychotherapy. Many evidence-based protocols for childhood diagnoses would benefit from parent education and coaching on helping their children implement certain recommendations. Take, for example, a child being treated for obsessive–compulsive disorder (OCD). Parents must play an integral part in their child's treatment by learning how to support them in incrementally facing their fears, rather than playing into the anxiety inherent in the diagnosis. Teaching parents why reassurance, a typically positive behavior, worsens the symptoms of OCD is an important part of the treatment for the child.

When you help the parent carry out a specific treatment protocol, you can follow these steps:

- Communicate with the child's individual therapist, unless you are providing parent guidance as part of child therapy. Find out what protocols the therapist is using so that you can assist the caregiver.
- Tailor the program you are using to the parent's skill level.
- When you suggest a self-help book or workbook—one example is *What to Do When You Worry Too Much* (Huebner, 2005)—work alongside the parent to guide them in how to use the resource.
- Explain psychological concepts in ways that can be helpful for parents. For example, grasping some cognitive-behavioral therapy (CBT) ideas, such as the impact of thoughts on feelings and the benefits of exposure, facing fears, and

shifting thoughts, facilitates treatment. You can teach psychological concepts, as appropriate, so that parents can reinforce the ideas in their children's work.

- Teach concepts from dialectical behavior therapy (DBT), such as the benefits of building interpersonal effectiveness and mindfulness skills as well as the benefits of radical acceptance and calming emotional distress (Linehan, 2014). These can be useful in a variety of circumstances. Parents often resonate with the DBT concept of "wise mind," which suggests that feelings and rational thoughts can come together to make more effective decisions.
- Describe concepts from trauma treatment, such as reexperiencing and dissociation, emotional reactions to trauma reminders, and unexpected behavioral responses, which may be important for parents to recognize.

Approaching Parent Guidance with a Nonjudgmental Stance

No child is born with an owner's manual and, in the same way that cars may operate differently, it is also true that children respond differently to interventions. Families may employ a variety of workable solutions. Despite the multiple ways to parent, some people judge parents for their choices and blame them for their children's misbehavior. Judgments arise when parents, professionals, and others scrutinize the parenting of people whose children behave poorly, not understanding that the solution this family has arrived at is the product of many previous trials. Some may privately, or not so privately, say that the issue is that the parents are not strict enough, are too strict, or do not have consistent rules or limits. They may discount the efforts of the parents, who likely are desperately trying to figure out the best interventions for their children, and ignore the impact of temperament, genetics, and life circumstances on behavior and mood. Parent guidance offers a unique opportunity, rarely afforded in the real world, to provide a blame-free zone in which to explore a variety of solutions.

EB had an experience during which she learned how blame and judgments about managing difficult child behavior can feel. Before finishing her doctoral degree, she was working as an assistant teacher for autistic children. The school planned a field trip to McDonald's for six nonverbal elementary-age children with autism. EB and her colleague thought this trip was a terrible idea, but were required by their superiors to make it happen. When they arrived at McDonald's, one of the children, nearly the same size as EB and lacking the skill to delay gratification, ran around grabbing french fries from the tables of the other customers. She took the child to the vestibule to prevent this behavior and to wait for her colleague, who now had the job of ordering the food for and managing five nonverbal children with autism. While EB waited for what seemed an eternity for the food to be ordered, many people judged her management of the situation. There was much unwelcome advice. The most persistent advice came from an older couple: "What if we gave him a shiny penny?" EB rejected their advice, which was delivered with good intentions and the strong belief that the shiny penny would have been an effective solution. She knew that this child would likely have eaten the shiny penny.

Many parents of challenging children are in exactly this situation all of the time; people offer advice that parents know from prior experience would not be successful. It helps to remember that sometimes behavior is very difficult to manage; that an inability to manage it may not be the fault of the person trying; that negative judgments when a parent is doing their best are unhelpful; and that problems are often predictable, if the target you set is unattainable (e.g., a successful trip to McDonald's for children who have difficulty waiting).

How Should Children Behave?

There are multiple viewpoints, in part culturally driven, regarding children's behavior and what level of obedience is reasonable and expectable. When the question "Should children behave?" is posed, the automatic response might be yes. However, it is a more nuanced question than that answer suggests. What level of obedience should be expected? Is it about thought-out expectations and values that parents have, or about what feels convenient and what parents have the energy to deal with? At what point can parental control become abusive? When is it neglectful to set no boundaries, expectations, or rules? How do "reasonable" parents behave? Can you help parents adjust their style to a combination of loving support and intentional choices about the family rules? As therapists, we need to know what we are comfortable with and come to an understanding of shared goals with families. Our therapy goals need to be co-created with parents, as most therapists will not accept a goal, for example, that a child must obey every command that is issued to them without questioning it, or a goal that a child's every whim and desire for comfort must be placated.

CASE STUDY: To Spank or Not to Spank?

A mother came in for help because her 3-year-old did not "behave." Specifically, the child did not listen to her mother and was therefore hard to control. Her mother noted that the child behaved much better with her father. The mother reported that her father spanked the girl, leading her to be "scared" of him. According to the mother, the father was not as concerned about his daughter's mental health and did not "believe" in therapy. The mother and the therapist had similar goals for the child's behavior, including improving behavior at home and in public, following directives, and having more enjoyable time with her parents. Through parent guidance, the mother and the therapist focused on learning techniques, including child-led play, identifying shared enjoyable activities, effective ways to set limits, and positive reinforcement for improved behavior. After completing her therapy, the mother had more parenting skills, which resulted in greater parenting satisfaction and an improved relationship with her daughter. The father observed the changes in his wife's relationship with their daughter, which enabled him to expand his repertoire beyond spanking and to seek similar improvements for his own relationship with their child.

Undoubtedly, there are some biases that impact this work that are harder than others to be aware of and acknowledge. In this case example, we are in favor of proactive interventions, while never promoting spanking as a method of behavior change. The preference for proactive interventions and the avoidance of corporal punishment that we, and many therapists doing this work, advocate are common. However, our preferred interventions are not universal. They may vary, depending on culture, subculture, and personal style. Our own upbringing, the subcultures within which we were raised, the broader cultural context, and what we learned through graduate school and ongoing clinical work, all play into our biases.

Our Approach

A transtheoretical approach, or one that integrates multiple theoretical orientations, provides therapists with a wider array of tools in working with varied families with unique presentations. We use this approach to parent guidance in this book, recognizing that "no one size fits all," and that having a foundation with an expansive toolkit will be of value both for graduate students at the start of their career and for long-practicing therapists. We also review intervention basics, including how relationships undergird interactions that form the bedrock of parent guidance work.

We favor a transtheoretical approach for a variety of reasons. Sometimes parents are reluctant to try a recommended intervention because it doesn't fit with their family culture or their skill set. At other times they believe that they have already tried what you are suggesting. In these situations, it is beneficial for the parent to have a variety of options for achieving the same outcome, as well as the skills to overcome barriers along the way. It is akin to choosing a different route when your GPS indicates heavy traffic or a road closure on the route you've chosen. Sometimes it takes longer than you would have originally hoped but it is faster, or more effective, than being in standstill traffic watching the aftereffects of a crash blocking the road.

PACT: A Strategy to Bring Together Many Approaches

In our integrative parent guidance work, we use the acronym "PACT" as our framework for boosting treatment effectiveness with caregiver intervention.

- **P (Partner).** Partnering is about the recognition of the critical relationships involved in helping parents and their children when they are struggling with mental health concerns. We see ourselves as partners with the parents who will carry out the interventions or modify their behavior to achieve an improvement. Developing a strong relationship with the parents or caregivers will result in impactful treatment.

- **A (Assess).** We view assessment broadly, in the sense that understanding as much of the problem and its context as possible is essential for developing and choosing an optimal treatment plan. Assessment is more than identifying a single problem. Instead, it is a process of developing a complete understanding of a child and the caregivers within the family context. Far too often a narrow path is chosen in child psychotherapy, in which the parents come in, name a problem, and a behavior plan is developed and implemented. Although both of us as therapists have developed plans involving rewards, we do so after completely evaluating the presenting problem and its context.

- **C (Choose).** Choosing how much parent involvement and which intervention(s) with particular aregivers makes sense is the next step in the process. Broadly this could entail deciding with whom to meet and how many times to meet with each person. Should the intervention be stand-alone parent guidance? If you will be the child's therapist, a key question may be how much parent involvement there should be. In some cases, parent intervention may constitute most, if not all, of the work and in other cases it may be a very small portion of the work. Once parent guidance is determined to be a useful intervention, there are a number of paths and tools to choose from. We delve into the choices for intervention and the elements that factor into decision making about the choice.

- **T (Treat** and evaluate outcomes). Once you have created a healthy working partnership with the family (P); assessed the child, family, and situation (A); and chosen

Partner

- "Have I made a connection with the caregiver?"
- "Do they seem to feel comfortable in session, even when disagreeing or asking questions?"

Assess

- "Do I understand the caregiver, the problem, the situation, and the relationship between the caregiver and child in order to choose an appropriate intervention?"
- "Do I have a working formulation of this child and family? "

Choose

- "Do I have a sense of whether parent guidance is appropriate and, if so, whether it should be incorporated into the child's treatment as an adjunct or whether it should be a stand-alone service?"
- "What intervention(s) do I think will be most helpful?"
- "Does the caregiver understand and agree, or buy in, to that idea?"

Treat and monitor progress

- "How will I move forward with treatment?"
- "How will I know if I am making progress?"
- "What are the likely obstacles to advancing?"
- "Do I need to troubleshoot and/or shift gears?"
- "What would signal a time to conclude this treatment?"
- Transition out of treatment

FIGURE INTRO.1. PACT checklist.

to use parent guidance (C); you can begin the treatment and monitoring-of-progress phase (T). The checklist in Figure Intro.1 may be helpful as you implement PACT with caregivers.

A Note on Terminology, Sources, and Bias

Terminology

Language is not neutral. To clarify our use of terms, there are words we use interchangeably, although they do not have exactly the same meaning. We use both *parent* and *caregiver* to identify the person with whom you are working. This person might be a biological parent, adoptive parent, or stepparent, or might be another member of the child's kin, such as a grandparent, aunt, uncle, or older sibling, now in the parenting role. The person might be a foster parent or a biological parent who does not currently have custody of the child. There are many ways people care for children, and we intend to leave no one out. We would also like to explicitly acknowledge and recognize that there are many kinds of family constellations. We see two-parent families, single-parent families, and families in which the two parents have separated and each spouse has a new partner who is involved in the raising of the child. We also see families with multiple parents in the household.

We welcome the diverse families that come to our offices. There can be racial or ethnic diversity, diversity regarding sexual orientation or gender identity, and socioeconomic or religious diversity. However, diversity can also occur in the context of values and expectations. Sometimes we make erroneous assumptions about the parents' reactions based on our biases. Early in her career, EB encountered an 8-year-old boy with medical trauma. His parents needed help in coaching him through a series of rectal exams. Over the course of the treatment, EB discovered that the school, noting the child's academic struggles, wished to retain him in the second grade. Heartbroken for the parents, EB dreaded speaking with them about this topic. When she brought it up, both parents smiled and told her that they thought it was a great idea, as it had been helpful for both of them early on in elementary school. We hope to keep an open mind to the different perspectives parents have.

We use the terms *parent guidance* and *parent coaching* interchangeably. Use whichever term feels more comfortable for you. We also use many words to refer to you, the parent guidance expert, including *provider, clinician,* and *therapist*. They are meant to imply the same role: a professional helper for parents.

Sources of Our Ideas

We have included many ideas that we hope you will find useful, but we cannot take credit for developing all of them. Our sources for ideas are derived from our years of clinical work and also from the classes, written resources, trainings, supervisors, supervisees, colleagues, and the families we have met. Where there was a reference to include, we did. Where there was not, please remember that a team of individuals co-created these ideas. The case material presented in this book consists of composite examples based on real patients whose identifying features are either changed or omitted. As a result of the fictionalization, confidentiality has not been breached.

Acknowledging Our Own Biases

While we present a transtheoretical approach, in that we advocate no single technique, we recognize that we frame the material within the particular lenses of our own professional and personal experiences. We have a strong attachment lens, prioritizing the relationship between the caregiver and child. Our philosophy, while attachment oriented, is predicated on our strong belief in two major concepts: that children benefit from parental structure, expectations, and love; and that skills are built in the context of opportunities and challenges rather than on easy paths which provide less possibility of learning.

Prioritizing both relationships and opportunities for growth fits within the framework of our personal and family cultures. Both of us were raised in the northeastern part of the United States with high academic and behavioral expectations. We grew up with a focus on critical thinking and a certain level of child autonomy. Families may have different parenting values and beliefs than we do. We try, throughout this book, to consciously recognize our biases to the extent that we can.

PART I

Foundations of Parent Guidance

This part addresses what you, as the clinician, need to know before beginning interventions. It helps you understand the factors contributing to how and why people parent the way they do, why attachment is the lens through which we approach parent guidance work, how to assess a variety of factors that may impact the symptom picture, and the importance of a strong working relationship with the caregivers. These understandings comprise the footing upon which you build your interventions.

CHAPTER 1

Contributors to Parenting Patterns

"I can't go anywhere with my daughter. I can't manage her behavior in public, and all of my relatives have something to say about me being too lenient or something. I'm sick of it. They have no idea what it is like to raise my daughter."

"We are applying to preschools for my son. If he does not get into a good one, this will set the trajectory for his whole education."

"I am from Jamaica, and my wife is from Australia. We are trying to raise a Black son in the United States."

"My parents drank. When they got angry, things got ugly. I don't ever want to act like that with my kids but I can't set limits."

"Generally I can manage my anxiety, but when it comes to my kids it really gets the best of me. I don't let them do a lot of things other kids do because I am too nervous."

Anxiety, limit setting, hopes and dreams, pressures, and disappointment. These are all part of normative parenting. They are also aspects of the work we do. We have seen all of the concerns raised in this list and many others. As parent guidance experts, we will parse out what is getting in the way of effective parenting. To do this, we need to understand patterns and contributors to the ongoing caregiving relationship.

Process and Patterns in the Parenting Relationship

The cornerstone of our work is the relationship between a caregiver and child: the patterns, process, and sets of rules that govern the relationship rather than the content of a specific interaction. There are few definitive best-parenting policies or specific musts or must nots. Relationships are about the totality of interactions, not just one: A strong parent–child relationship can withstand many missteps.

We have worked with many parents who sheepishly report that they did something they were not proud of with their child and wonder what damage this incident (often yelling at the child in a moment of anger) has done. We remind them that their relationship with their child is about long-standing patterns, and this one instance will not be the undoing of a generally strong relationship. As we consider how someone engages in this broad group of activities that we have dubbed "parenting," we need to focus on general patterns and use specific examples as just that: examples, or hypothesis generators, and teachable moments. Even Baumrind's (1971) parenting styles were about just that: styles, not specific behaviors. Her authoritative parenting style, with high levels of structure as well as high levels of support and warmth, was deemed optimal. This does not mean that every interaction between the caregiver and child is characterized by both high structure as well as warmth. Instead, we are hoping for trends in interactions that the child can generally count on to occur in a certain way. There is predictability not so much about the specifics, but about the typical ways of being together.

For example, think about a mother picking her daughter up from school. The daughter walks over to the car with a friend and asks the mother, in front of the friend, whether the friend can come over to play. The mother says yes but feels uncomfortable about the position her daughter put her in. At a later time, the mother explains that asking in front of the friend is inappropriate, as it puts her in a challenging situation during which she feels uncomfortable responding negatively. This mother has many choices about how to handle the situation. She does not embarrass or yell at the daughter, instead waiting to impart the lesson. She does, however, set a limit. This daughter can likely count on her mother to behave in ways consistent with this interchange. The daughter will not expect to be embarrassed by her mother, or yelled at, nor will she expect that anything goes. Within that framework, the specifics of their interactions can vary but, barring other circumstances or vulnerability factors, there is a certain basic style of interaction that can be anticipated.

Internal characteristics, familial patterns, societal forces, and individual experiences all influence these patterns that we see. Practitioners are expected to be conscious of many factors and circumstances that play into the presentations we see in our offices. The current state of clinical practice requires clinicians to be aware of such factors as the possibility of trauma and the need for trauma-informed care, the likelihood that abuse of an opioid or other drug may have touched this family, or the likelihood that there are LGBTQIA+ issues at play, to name some of them.

Understanding the Parent's World

Though it is beyond the scope of this book to review all of the cultures you will encounter, it is important to inquire about the circumstances of the parents you help. When working with families from any background different from your own, pay attention to the very real values and concerns that influence parenting behaviors. Some families want to ensure the transmission of cultural values that may differ from the dominant culture. Others struggle as a result of to a lack of privilege or lack of resources. For example, families of color may feel the need to impart information to their offspring about ways to behave in order to keep their child safe in the world.

In order to provide culturally responsive care, as the parent guidance expert:

- Be aware of your own values and beliefs. Learn about the culture of your patient families, considering culture in the broadest sense. Worksheet 1.1, "Know Your Values as a Parent Guidance Expert," at the end of the chapter, helps clarify these values.
- Educate yourself about how racial, ethnic, and cultural identity and issues play into psychotherapy (Sue et al., 2019; Hays & Erford, 2017).
- Consider that your own beliefs and values may be influencing your interventions as much as your education on best practices.
- When you are concerned about a cultural or values mismatch, ask the family for more information or seek information from a knowledgeable outside source.
- Seek consultation or supervision when you are unsure.

Awareness of the stressors that a caregiver contends with helps you in planning parent guidance interventions. Some of the outside sources of these stressors may include schools and protective service agencies. Expectations from schools, such as homework, special projects, and family involvement, add to the demands on a parent. One parent we know, when faced with an unreasonable demand regarding his daughter's school project, told his daughter's teacher, "I have already passed third grade. I am not going to do this project." This overstressed parent did not feel that his child's project, which relied heavily on parental involvement, was a good use of his time and energy. Families struggling with fewer resources may have limited time and energy for our interventions.

Whether or not protective services are involved with a family may also impact someone's parenting. In many subcultures and socioeconomic echelons, protective services are an ever-present concern, with the possibility of being reported weighing on families, simply because they have seen it happen to families they know. This unintended presence sometimes keeps parents from seeking help or from being fully honest once they are in therapy. Caregivers may avail themselves of your services as a clinician, willingly or out of necessity, because of requirements imposed upon them by protective services. When this is the case, you must work with them to attain some level of engagement.

Pressures Facing Parents Today

Pressure exerted by others can make it challenging to listen to one's own parenting instincts, and many parents are really good at defining "shoulds" for themselves: "As a parent I should do this and I should do that." JDS works with one parent who is so good at telling herself what she should be doing that they have dubbed it her superpower. The mother has determined "shoulds" about what she does for her children that her children do not even agree with; they think she is a great parent, but she does an excellent job of convincing herself that she has not done enough for them.

Pressures from both internal and external sources impact parenting and therefore children. Our own awareness of these concerns, as parent coaches, allows us to raise the questions and help caregivers determine what is helpful and what they can let go of.

Shoulds may feel similar to values or may disguise themselves as values. Values have to do with one's principles and standards, what an individual considers to be important. Shoulds have more to do with expectations and judgments than with values but are not necessarily tied to priorities, standards, or principles.

Some internal pressures, though, are connected to values. Do not assume that you know what a caregiver's values are, as they can be different than what you might expect. Consider that one mother may value her children seeing her as a working mother. The same mother may also be self-critical because she is working and not able to provide freshly baked snacks when her children arrive home from school every day. These values are in conflict and cause some distress. Many parents, especially mothers, are compared to the impossible ideal of "supermom/superparent" by themselves and others, providing another source of distress.

In addition, for many parents getting daily tasks completed can be challenging. It is often quicker and easier for a parent to complete daily tasks instead of allowing the time for their child to develop the skills. It greases the wheels and allows the family to function more smoothly. However, taking over these tasks may not develop the independence in their child that the parent eventually hopes for. Think about why family members do what they do.

Some Parenting Styles

What does parenting today look like? It depends on the parent. We identify and discuss some of the parenting styles you may see. Think about whether these parenting styles help the child develop the skills and values that their caregiver is trying to inspire.

The Very Involved Parent

New terms, such as *snowplow* and *helicopter* parents, have been coined to describe parents whose behavior indicates a need to protect their children from danger or from missing out. Snowplow parents clear the way so that their children have an easy path forward. Helicopter parents hover and swoop in to take care of any difficulty as it arises. The potential reasons for this behavior include anxiety, concern for their children, the desire for their children to succeed, and the difficulty of tolerating their children's pain or discomfort.

Trying to Encourage More Independence

There is a movement for "free-range" parenting, as described by Lenore Skenazy (2009). Her book's subtitle is *Giving Our Children the Freedom We Had Without Going Nuts with Worry.* It involves encouraging developmentally appropriate independence and accepting a higher level of parental risk. This concept runs counter to what we often see in parenting involvement and may challenge our own level of comfort with risk.

Focusing on Achievement and Future Success

Preparation H is the colloquial term for a parenting style in which the parent is trying to prepare their child for Harvard University or some other prestigious institution of higher education. Parents gear much of their parenting energy to helping their child be competitive for college entry. This style may also be promoted by their child's school explicitly or more subtly pervade the culture of a "good" school system. Children who are raised with "Preparation H" are overscheduled with extracurricular activities to improve their chances for future success. While they may be expected to be leaders in school and excel in music or sports, they often have strikingly few responsibilities at home in order to manage their commitments. JDS has had many conversations with parents about managing what they recognize as the compulsion to ensure that their children have a competitive edge. Even though they recognize the compulsive quality of what they are doing, many of these same parents create as many opportunities as possible for their child in order to add items to their résumés and college applications.

Tiger Parents

A subtype of the achievement-oriented parent is the "Tiger Mom." This descriptor became well known when Amy Chua published her book *Battle Hymn of the Tiger Mother* in 2011. By her own description, a tiger mother raises her children in a strict and traditionally Chinese way, encouraging achievement at high levels and discouraging social engagement. Descriptions of parenting moments in this book may be challenging for Western readers. However, Chua's view of her strategy as superior, mostly as evidenced by the success of the children she describes, may have more appeal to your patients than you realize.

Children as Equal Partners

Different regions and places may have different ideas about what is good parenting. Cambridge, Massachusetts, where EB lives, has a reputation for lenient parenting in what is known as "the Cambridge parenting style." In this style, which has become something of a stereotype and exaggerated, children are treated as equals, with preschoolers weighing in on parental decisions about everything from dinner menus to family scheduling and beyond. Logical reasoning and intellectual dialogue are seen as important skills to inculcate in the very young. Children are also idealized, in the sense that many behaviors that would be seen as misbehaviors in other cultures are viewed as charming. Once a child unknown to EB joined her table at a restaurant when she was eating with friends and ate off their plates. The child's parents smiled as though this behavior would be an enjoyable treat for us. In this situation, the parents did not set limits, nor did they view this conduct as inappropriate.

Attachment Parenting

There are many parenting issues that spark strong opinions and feelings and may be tied to closely held values. Some of these issues include co-sleeping and breast-feeding and are sometimes related to a focus on the importance of "attachment parenting" (Sears & Sears, 2001), which is a style of parenting thought to promote attachment between the parent and child. This language is used in the lay literature and is differentiated from the attachment styles and influences that we refer to when discussing attachment research literature. You, the clinician, may also have strong feelings about attachment parenting. Be mindful of what is helpful for the family, what falls within your purview, what information is available in the scholarly literature (e.g., Bar et al., 2016, on the benefits of breast-feeding, and McKenna & McDade, 2005, on the benefits of co-sleeping), and what represents a clash of values if there is one.

How Does This Knowledge of Parenting Styles Impact Your Work?

Your clinical skills, accumulated best practices, and creative ideas—along with your background and values—will be combined with what you know about families and how to approach them. These are all factors that you bring into the therapy space. The parents with whom you work will have their own values and background and their practices and experiences from their day-to-day world. Your job involves recognizing how all of them combine to effect positive change with families.

The Importance of Understanding Attachment in Parent Guidance

Although the early relationship between parent and infant is affected by what each one contributes (Sameroff, 2009), it is up to the parent to lay the groundwork for both parent and child to function effectively. Think about attachment as a stage play. The caregiver is responsible for creating the sets, making the costumes, booking the theater, and developing the basic plot lines. Both the parent and the child play a role, and both will develop lines, deliver them in certain ways, and perhaps improvise new ones. With both parent and child playing their parts, it becomes a drama that could not happen without both actors, but much of the production relies on the caregiver.

The Importance of Early Interactions and Relationships for Life Outcomes

A few basic principles are essential for the practitioner of parent guidance to understand in order to provide quality care. Essentially, early interactions with parents form the foundation of how children see the world, interact with others, deal with emotions, and understand how relationships are conducted.

In referring to attachment and attachment theory, we are talking about the relationship patterns that develop in the relationship between caregivers and their children.

Mary Ainsworth and colleagues' seminal book *Patterns of Attachment* (1978) highlights the concept that interactions are not unique events, but rather that they flow from patterns developed over time. Ainsworth describes three patterns of infant behavior, one of which classifies infants as "secure" when they seek comfort from the parent, prefer the parent to a stranger, express feelings, and explore new environments in their parent's presence. With healthy caregivers, children's basic needs as well as their need for consistency, care, soothing, connection, attunement, and help with emotion regulation are met.

In parent guidance, we are often helping parents learn to provide these basic skills so that their children develop a sense of security, a base from which to explore their world, ways to express a range of emotions and needs, and the ability to self-regulate.

How Caregivers Parent May Reflect How They Were Parented

The way that the caregiver parents has a lot to do with their own early attachment. Their attachment style, developed in part through repeated interactions with their own caregiver, will affect their own emotion regulation as well as how they relate to those close to them, including their children. People learn to parent first and foremost by having been parented. This early relationship with their own caregivers may be the driving force behind their own relationships, interaction style, affect management, and parenting practices (Posada et al., 2002; Sroufe et al., 2005).

The caregivers' ability to be responsive to their children varies, and that variability is, to a significant extent, related to their own ideas of what it means to be a parent, otherwise known as their internal working model of caregiving (Main et al., 1985). When Roy Muir says, in the influential therapy film *When the Bough Breaks* that "people think parenting comes naturally," he points out that it does come naturally but not necessarily how you wish it to.

In reacting to their experiences in their families of origin, some parents behave similarly to their own caregivers, whereas others will actively try to do things differently, as in Judith Siegel's (2004) concept of "dis-identification." Both of these strategies, repeating patterns or actively trying to do something different, are about the parents' early histories and are not necessarily a good match for the child or the situation. There is evidence that a careful consideration of childhood relationships in young adulthood leads to improved parenting (Shlafer et al., 2015). One key to adjusting parenting, in the context of parent guidance, is to think actively about how a caregiver parents in relation to their own early experiences.

CASE STUDY: History of Trauma in the Caregiver

Consider this stark example. A clinician was providing parent guidance as an adjunct to her work with an 8-year-old boy. The parents had lost custody when a teacher reported finding bruises on the boy. After a year in foster care, the boy was reunited with his biological family. The therapist focused on helping the boy readjust to life at home with his biological parents, especially given his feelings about the earlier physical abuse that had occurred.

The parent guidance part was more difficult. In meeting alone with the parents, the therapist was able to get a better sense of where they were coming from. In reviewing their childhood history, she discovered that these caregivers had also experienced significant childhood trauma. One of them had so many scars on her body that she was too ashamed to go to the doctor. With this information, the clinician targeted her interventions differently. Bringing this information into the open allowed the caregivers to link their own childhoods to their current parenting struggles. They developed a more conscious recognition of the impact their upbringing had on their parenting and were able to use this insight to work on changing their behavior. Understanding the caregivers' stories with regard to family of origin, attachment, and trauma allowed the parents to develop, with the therapist's help, more healthy patterns with their own children going forward.

Use Worksheet 1.2, "What Kind of Parenting Did I Have?," at the end of the chapter, to help parents think about the parenting they experienced and how it may impact the way they are raising their child.

Using Your Understanding of Attachment in Parent Guidance Work

Your knowledge of attachment needs to be integrated into your consultation with caregivers. A primary goal of parent guidance will often be to improve the relationship between parent and child and to enhance their working alliance. Often the parent and child are frustrated with each other and feel that something is not working in their relationship. If we are able to improve parent–child attachment as part of our parent guidance work, we will be leaving an indelible mark on the life of a child.

The work goes beyond just "skills building." Evidence has shown that focusing on improving the attachment between parent and child is more effective in treatment for maltreated preschoolers than building parenting skills alone (Toth et al., 2002). When parents relate more positively with their children, they stand a better chance of effectively teaching their children about the emotional world (Newland & Crnic, 2011). And when children are comforted by parents, they learn self-regulation (Cole et al., 2009; Sroufe et al., 2005). Attachment patterns that are developed early on continue to impact relationships, including romantic relationships and relationships with one's children (e.g., Raby et al., 2015; Scharff et al., 2004). So when thinking about attachment style, think not only about the child's attachment style, but also about the parent's attachment style, what the parent's attachment to their parents looks like, and what the couple's (if there is one) attachment to each other looks like.

The Transactional Nature of the Caregiving Relationship

Interactions between the caregiver and child change both individuals, as described by Sameroff's transactional model (2009), mentioned earlier in this chapter. Who the child is will impact the nature of the parenting, as it is an inherently reciprocal and transactional relationship in which both parties are changed. For example, we know a parent who never planned to co-sleep. She believed it would be a hard habit to break, which led to her decision not to try it. Then she had a child who really struggled with sleep, and it was exhausting. Suddenly she was co-sleeping!

A parent may intend to have many rules, but finds that their child is more cautious and needs little imposed structure. Another caregiver may have a laid-back style, but then have a child who benefits from more structure. These examples describe situations in which a parent may make a conscious decision to adjust their style to meet the needs of the child. However, perhaps more often, the transactions between the parent and child will alter the style of the parent without that caregiver making a conscious decision. A colicky infant may prove frustrating for the caregiver, who may feel that, no matter what they try, they are often not able to soothe their child. The parent will find that their efforts are not reinforced the way they would be with another child. Eventually they may put in less effort to soothe the child and unknowingly become surlier in their interactions.

What Is the Job of a Parent?

What do we consider to be the basic job of a parent? How, as parent guidance consultants, do we help people manage the occupation of "parent" when the job is more difficult than the one they applied for? The Australian government (NSW Government, n.d.) defined the job of parent as being to "protect your child from harm, to provide your child with food, clothing, and a place to live, to financially support your child, to provide safety, supervision and control, to provide medical care, and to provide an education." Beyond these basic requirements, we would add that a parent's job is to create an environment in which children can thrive; feel loved; have opportunities to grow, develop, and explore; understand reasonable boundaries and behaviors; and rely on their secure attachment relationship (as described by Bowlby, 1988).

As exemplified in Australia's list of parental responsibilities, parents do not need to be perfect. They need to be "good enough." Caregivers are not evaluated based on whether they get an A in parenting. In fact, they are typically "evaluated" as parents only when something problematic shows up on the radar.

Approach parent guidance work thinking about your limited time with the parents and the practical and emotional resources they have to make changes. You will have many ideas to suggest to caregivers, but you will not throw everything at them at once. Your goal will not be to immediately solve every issue, work on every skill, and teach every technique. It is not about developing elaborate rules and behavioral systems. It is instead about shifting patterns in small increments to be more effective and positive. Your goal may be just to help families make enough change, one step at a time, to improve their quality of life.

WORKSHEET 1.1

Know Your Values as a Parent Guidance Expert

It may be useful to bring yourself back to the foundations of your parent guidance work. Thinking about your own experiences and values may help you understand your biases as well as what is important to you in supporting the caregivers with whom you work. There are no "right" answers.

- Why do I want to do parent guidance?
- What is my view about the role of a parent?
- What is an ideal parent?
- How do I view the balance of supporting children and building independence?
- If I have children, how did I raise them?
- What am I proud about in my parenting or in my time with children in my family?
- What do I wish I had done differently?
- If I don't have children, how would I raise them if I did?
- When families have different parenting values than I do, how do I manage the mismatch?
- How do I cope when other parents in my community have a difference of opinion?
- What do I get out of helping other people?
- Am I cooperative or competitive with others in the community as a parent?

How would I rate these parenting values on a scale of (1) not important to (5) very important?

____ warmth	____ teaching	____ playing	____ honesty
____ building character	____ openness	____ rules	____ obedience
____ love	____ forgiveness	____ structure	____ clarity
____ intergenerational contact	____ making money	____ discipline	____ being kind
____ preparing for college	____ parent's job/career	____ achievement in sports	____ achievement in music
____ achievement in arts	____ parent's relationship with partner	____ parent's need for nonparenting activities	____ achievement in school

WORKSHEET 1.2

What Kind of Parenting Did I Have?

The best things about how my parent raised me

The worst things about how my parent raised me

Things I am doing like my parent did

Things I am not doing like my parent did

Things I want to make sure I do

Things I want to make sure I don't do or do less

CHAPTER 2

Strategies for Partnering

Nurturing the Critical Relationships

Though the relationship between the parent and child is paramount, the relationship between the clinician and caregivers is critical for moving forward in parent guidance. Multiple studies identify the relationship or alliance with the client as a central component in all forms of psychotherapy (Falkenström et al., 2013; Feller & Cottone, 2012; Horvath, 2001). This alliance is equally important in parent guidance work, as the clinician needs to develop and maintain a trusting connection with the caregiver (Lieberman et al., 2019) in order to help them achieve their parenting goals. Keeping this connection requires attending to this relationship on an ongoing basis. "Attending to" is the active and intentional process of continuing to monitor and grow the therapeutic alliance, and repair any rifts as needed.

Even though the parents may not be the targeted patients or clients, we are expecting them to do very challenging work. It may involve examining their own moods, functioning, skills, patterns of behavior, and the attachment both to their child and potentially to their family of origin. We are asking caregivers to delve deep when they may have simply expected their child to come to therapy and "be fixed." Parents will be putting trust in you, the clinician, and investing time, energy, and effort into changing ingrained patterns of behavior and interactions with their child. Early in the process, you may find that they do not believe that this effort will pay off. Unlike you, they have not worked with many other families or had supervisors who could report years of experiences of success in similar circumstances. Hence, despite the caregiver not being the "identified patient," the same type of foundational relationship must exist with them as you would expect to have with any other client or patient.

PACT: "P" for "Partner"

Conceptualizing Your Role as a Consultant

Clinicians providing parent guidance are often serving in a consulting role. We can offer a range of options that we hope will be helpful, and parents can choose among them. We are listening and suggesting, not dictating. We have knowledge and experience that they do not have, but we are not imposing our decisions on them.

Involving All Relevant Caregivers

Frequently in child therapy or stand-alone parent coaching, the therapist winds up interfacing mostly with one parent: the parent who brings the child to treatment, often a mother. In stand-alone parent guidance, you may have the opportunity to work with two parents, although sometimes it is difficult to get all of the caregivers to an appointment. If only one parent is able to participate, you can still do good work with that person, but when all caregivers are included, and ideally working in sync, there is a greater likelihood of positive change. Hence, engaging fathers, who less often participate in the treatment, may be especially important. Other regular caregivers, such as nannies and grandparents, may also be involved. Understanding how each caregiver interacts with the child will provide fodder for therapeutic work.

When a relevant caregiver is not attending appointments, prioritize building that relationship in other ways. Reach out by phone. Let them know that you recognize that they play an important role in the child's life, and you would like to hear their opinion about the situation. They may be able to attend a session via a telehealth platform. If one caregiver is not able to attend because of practical constraints, or is unwilling to engage, continue the work with the presenting caregiver. That initial effort may open the door to future communication with the parent who does not participate.

A Comfortable and Open Stance

A trusting relationship provides the context and ballast for following the advice of the clinician. When a clinician recommends that the best way to help a child change is by changing parental behavior, this advice can understandably be heard by the parent as "This child's problem is your fault" or "If you were only a better caregiver your child would not have these problems." The thoughtful clinician conveys the utility of caregiver change without assigning blame or judgment.

For example, a mother of a toddler came in for an assessment. During the assessment she told the clinician that her child had violent tantrums that sometimes left him bruised, as he would flail around in small spaces and hit himself against objects. She had experienced very upsetting interactions in the local hospital emergency department because the staff appeared to believe that she was physically abusive. During one trip to the emergency department, the hospital staff reported her to child protective services. On a later visit to the hospital, the child had a tantrum *in* the emergency department. The staff treated her very differently after that incident.

While previously the hospital staff felt reasonably obligated to file a report with protective services, imagine how this mother felt when she was trying to get her child cared for and, instead, she was treated as the cause of harm. She worked successfully with the clinician on learning better ways to manage her child, who had a very difficult temperament. That work was doable because the mother felt understood from very early on in the therapy. The clinician conveyed to the mother that she believed her, educated her about temperament, and talked about what would likely be effective, given the child's nature. The mother knew that she was not being blamed and that she could effect change, and she felt empowered rather than embarrassed.

Fostering the Therapeutic Relationship

Hear the Parent's Story

The importance of an empathic stance cannot be overstated (Feller & Cottone, 2012). After the initial "handshake," whether literal or metaphorical, the clinician has the opportunity to hear the parent's story. This means not just *letting* the parent tell their story but really listening to and hearing it. The parent benefits from knowing that you, as the therapist, understand why they are where they are, why they are parenting the way they are, and what other struggles they are coping with. Listening is a harder skill to master than it seems at first. Active listening, which involves deep attention to another person's words as evidenced by interested body language, eye contact, and intense concentration, can be an effective intervention in itself (Kawamichi et al., 2014). It requires the listener to allow the speaker to continue speaking, despite the content perhaps not meeting the therapist's desire for focused information. In the first sessions with parents, active listening involves connecting and "sitting with" intense emotions, such as anxiety, distress, and regret. Seeking an understanding of the *why* behind a parenting style or behavior will allow you to be more empathic and provide an inroad to addressing the behavior. This is especially important, because if the therapist jumps in too hastily with interventions without a full understanding of the situation, the advice could be read as critical or off base.

In addition to *hearing* the parent's story *convey* to the parent that their story was heard and understood. Caregivers are more likely to listen and try what is suggested when they feel that their perspective has been heard. They are also more likely to be honest about their shortcomings and admit when they have not tried something, or when they did something they were trying not to do. Understanding the parent's story, motivations, and other factors leading to their behavior also helps us target interventions appropriately and usefully.

Acknowledge that caregivers are working hard already, and that therapy will take more hard work. One of the dialectics discussed in dialectical behavior therapy (DBT) is the notion that people are doing the best that they can and also that they still have to do better (Linehan, 1993). Both can be true at the same time, and this fact can be communicated effectively to the parents. Parenting is hard work and is even more difficult for people who do not have strong skills in this area or who have children with mental health and behavioral concerns. Communicate that you are there to help; they are not in this venture alone.

Tone and Word Choice

It is important to remember that using a nonjudgmental tone conveys empathy, as can word choice. Empathy can also be conveyed through active listening, validation, and reflection. Sometimes clinicians know the reasons for a constellation of behaviors, but fail to indicate that they "get" where the person is coming from. The difference between "I understand the reason" and "I get it" is big and is felt by the parents.

CASE STUDY: Tolerating Parent Anger

A supervisee once reported that a parent was angry with her. The supervisee felt the mother was not being reasonable, because she believed she had addressed the mother's concerns. As the tale unfolded, it was clear that the mother was upset with one of the clinician's comments. In response to the anger, the clinician explained her reasoning in a very neutral way. Since her reasons made sense, the clinician thought the mother should be able to hear them and move on. She approached the mother with the statement "I can see why you felt that way but . . ." in a matter-of-fact tone that came across as dismissive. She did not address the mother's affect and therefore inadvertently communicated that she was not understanding where the mother was coming from at all, despite stating "I can see why you felt that way." What was meant to be a relationship repair became an additional relational breach. The clinician's effort to approach the mother's anger by focusing on the content of the words rather than on the tone of the message backfired, leading to an empathic failure. In supervision the clinician recognized that it was her own frustration and discomfort with the mother's expressed feelings that led her to approach the situation this way.

Parents who have felt judged in the past or who have had negative experiences with various agencies and systems may have an understandably heightened sensitivity to tone and word choice. It is worth asking specifically about experiences with previous therapists, agencies, schools, and other systems, paying attention to what the parents felt worked well and what did not. While you may ultimately choose similar interventions, you will be able to be more mindful of how you implement them, in part based on this information. Positive tones and messages, when relevant to the situation, can go a long way in establishing and maintaining the partnering relationship with the caregiver.

Positive Responses and Normalizing

Encouragement and cheerleading related to parental effort are useful even when the parent has not been "perfect" in their reactions to their child's behavior. Sometimes positive feedback can be even more powerful when the parent is struggling to prioritize the child's needs. When it makes sense, normalize parental reactions even when they are not ideal but reflect the caregiver's reasonable experience as a person as well as a parent. The following scenario is one example.

Caregiver: (*sheepishly*) I lost it with my kid yesterday.

Therapist: Tell me what happened.

Caregiver: He is constantly losing things. I know it's because of his ADHD [attention-deficit/hyperactivity disorder] and I try to do what I can but sometimes I just lose it. He lost the third pair of headphones I've gotten him this school year. He needs them for school, and he has to bring them back and forth. So he got in the car after school and realized he didn't have them. He had no idea where they were. I was just angry. I started yelling at him. He wound up feeling really badly and crying. It wasn't helpful. I felt terrible. It didn't solve the problem.

THERAPIST: That sounds like it is pretty frustrating. You get that he is doing the best he can but that doesn't solve the problem.

CAREGIVER: Yeah.

THERAPIST: Do you know any parents who never yell at their kids?

CAREGIVER: No.

THERAPIST: I know you would prefer it if you always kept your cool and responded to him in calm and productive ways, but I am not sure that it is realistic to think you can do that every single time. Parents sometimes yell at their kids.

Create Space for Voicing Negative Feelings about the Child

Some of the most challenging conversations with parents have to do with how they feel about their children. Sometimes parents reveal a dislike of their child or their regret about having a child. Some may even feel that they do not love their child. It is powerful for a parent to bravely admit that they do not feel about their child the way they think they should. One way to broach this topic could be as follows:

THERAPIST: I want to bring up something that may be hard to talk about.

CAREGIVER: (*tentatively*) Okay.

THERAPIST: One of the things that can be really hard for parents to admit is that they don't enjoy their child. Some parents don't like their child, but feel that they don't want to say so out loud. I wanted to check in about how you are feeling about Bella. This is a good space to address all sorts of feelings.

CAREGIVER: This is really hard. Everyone is supposed to love their child more than anything in the world.

THERAPIST: We can talk about what's real, not just what is "supposed to be."

CAREGIVER: Well, when we had her, we had this image of what raising a kid would be like. We knew it would be hard but she's been really hard. She's just mean. At this point, I don't even know if I love her. I can't believe I am saying this out loud!

THERAPIST: I understand. This is really not how you thought things would go.

CAREGIVER: Nope! She never cuddled. She's been difficult since the beginning. I've really had it.

Therapist: Can we work on finding ways for you to enjoy each other? Let's think about small changes to start. It's going to take some work.

Caregiver: Okay, if you think it's possible.

Address negative feelings about the child in an open and accepting manner. Sometimes these feelings progress into a sense of guilt, and sometimes they do not. We can have very honest and difficult conversations with parents about their feelings regarding their children. Remember though to encourage this conversation without the child present if you are also the child's therapist. For most evaluations of children, it is important to schedule a portion of the assessment with the parent alone, so that these feelings can be appropriately aired. Then difficult comments and feelings can be addressed, and you can assess whether adding parent guidance to joint therapy or scheduling standalone parent guidance would be beneficial. It is not therapeutic for children to hear their parents rattle off a litany of complaints about them. They may hear complaints about their behavior frequently at home, and one intervention could be educating the caregiver about helpful ways and contexts in which to vent about the child that will not worsen the situation or create negative self-feelings in the child.

Use the Parents' Names

Ask the parents how they prefer to be addressed. Calling them by their correct last name, with a favored title (i.e., Ms., Mrs., Dr., Mr., Mx.), or by their first name, is preferable to calling them Mom or Dad, which could suggest that you do not remember their name, do not see them as individuals aside from their relationship with their child, or are very casual in your manner. Many clinicians have the habit of saying, "What do you think, Mom?" as if the parent were the clinician's mother. It is reasonable, however, in front of their child, to refer to them as "your mom" or "your dad."

Figure 2.1 summarizes the main points we have covered so far.

Moving from Relationship Building to Intervening

You may wonder when the therapist can move from developing the partnering relationship, or building rapport, to intervening. The answer is that you are working on building rapport, performing an assessment, and finding ways to intervene from the first interaction.

Establishing a Therapeutic Contract

A "therapeutic contract" with a parent is not a formal written agreement that both parties have signed. Rather, it means that you have explicitly or implicitly agreed on what to work on to achieve desired change. As treatment continues, it implies that you are still working together toward shared goals. Use the relationship to co-create and

Key Points to Remember and Utilize, Especially in Early Sessions

Active listening and empathy involve:

- Listening
- Positive and open body language
- Eye contact
- Not interrupting
- Mirroring/reflection
- Validating statements that convey that a message has been heard
- Nonjudgmental stance

Measure rapport by observing the parents, including:

- Nonverbal cues
- Verbal cues
- Response to therapist suggestions or questions
- Mood

FIGURE 2.1. Building your partnership: Fostering relationships with caregivers.

determine strategies, allowing for an open dialogue about what is helping. When the caregiver shows enthusiasm or renewed hope or makes an effort toward reaching discussed goals, you have a sense that you are moving forward. You may get "I'm not sure about that but I'm willing to give it a try" rather than enthusiasm, but that is enough to start with. Alternately, quizzical looks and noncommittal utterances, or multiple sessions during which you feel that you are working hard but the parent is not communicate that you need to revisit the treatment plan.

Breaches in the Alliance

Parent guidance therapy may continue smoothly, or there may be hiccups along the way. Attend to these hiccups, paying special attention to whether there has been a breach in the therapeutic alliance. There are cues as to when such a rift occurs, which can range from caregivers not responding as openly or positively to statements in session, to actively appearing angry, to caregivers not practicing between sessions as discussed, to caregivers not coming to sessions as expected.

A variety of situations may lead to a rupture in the relationship. Examples could include filing a report of abuse or neglect, a time when the parent felt that you ignored what they tried to convey or did not understand how challenging the situation was for them, or simply saying something that offended them. These incidents do not imply that therapy has come to an end. They may, however, signify that active repair work needs to happen. You can do this work by being empathic and unafraid, listening and talking about the difficult circumstance. Impart how important this conversation is and how much you appreciate the caregiver engaging in it with you.

> **CASE STUDY: A Therapy Repair**
>
> A mother called the clinician working with her adolescent child. She was upset about something the youth had done and was close to tears. During the conversation, the therapist used humor, as she sometimes does. She made a joke about a way the mother could cope with the distressing situation that she assumed the mother understood as a recognition of how distressing the situation was rather than as a literal suggestion. Several days later the mother asked for a conversation. She conveyed to the therapist that this comment offended her. The therapist apologized, explained that she intended to use humor to help the mother cope with the situation, and actively listened to the mother's concerns. This repair with the therapist was possible because of the strong foundational relationship that had been established, allowing the mother to express her concerns explicitly. By having the conversation, the partnering was reestablished and treatment continued.

Even in the absence of partnering ruptures, check in with the caregiver about the therapeutic alliance (Slone & Owen, 2015) and their assessment of progress.

Managing Yourself in the Parent Guidance Relationship

Treating Parents as You Wish They Would Treat Their Children

According to Tracey and colleagues (2012), the parallel process is a phenomenon in which interaction patterns are replicated, such as when the therapist treats the parent as the parent treats the child. When you partner well with the parent, you model respect and collaboration. For example, if the parent confesses that they did something you had suggested they not do, respond to them with the openness you would want them to show toward their children. Let them know that it was helpful that they told you, and that you can work together on figuring out how to do things differently in the future.

Similarly, we ask parents to develop attunement to what their child is experiencing and communicating even when they make mistakes. Again, for the therapist, demonstrating attunement can be useful, both for the sake of modeling itself so that the caregiver can experience what it feels like and how helpful it is, but also because adults (like children) do not always clearly communicate what they are feeling and why.

Managing Your Own Feelings

Therapists will have periods of feeling frustrated with the caregivers with whom they are working in the same way that parents feel frustrated with their children. Parents do not always implement suggested strategies, even when we believe they are necessary, such as empathizing with their child or completing homework agreed to in session. Parents become frustrated with their child when they are not responding in the expected way. The therapist, in turn, may regard the parent in the same way as the parent regards the child. When this happens, the therapist, though frustrated, can respond to the parent as we wish the parent would respond to the child. Use this parallel process to become more attuned to what is happening in the therapy. A parent who is difficult to work with is likely the parent who most needs therapeutic support.

Attend to these feelings for multiple reasons. Negative feelings toward a client can impact the work you do. These feelings may also help you gauge the relationship with the parent. If you are feeling angry or uncomfortable, what is the likelihood that they are also having negative feelings about the relationship with you? Is it time to revisit the partnering aspect of the PACT framework? Parent guidance can be especially evocative for therapists who know that children are suffering when their parents are not behaving optimally. Use consultation and supervision to check on and better understand these reactions. Keep the focus on helping the child and on doing what will achieve that goal.

Conveying Expertise versus Being the Expert

Parents choose to work with you because they expect that you have the knowledge and skills to help them. Conveying expertise while partnering with a parent, who knows their child best, can be challenging. Caregivers will value different aspects of your experience: For some people, expertise involves degrees and credentials, including such things as where you went to graduate school and where your training occurred. Others will ask about your experience working with families or your personal status as a parent. You do not have to be a parent to do parent guidance or to convey confidence in your ability to do so. Your goal will be to use your expertise to both build the partnering relationship and to provide support that will guide the way.

Another point to keep in mind is that, although parents choose a therapist to access their expertise, the power differential between the therapist and the client can cause difficulty (De Varis, 1994). There is a difference between claiming the power of the expert role, and having valued expertise that is clinically useful. Therapists have knowledge and experience (Hill et al., 2017), but problems can arise when they "jump in" with their advice too soon, ignoring the knowledge that parents have. When this happens, therapists miss the nuanced understanding of the child's circumstances, stressors, and patterns that parents have gained over the years and the previous interventions that parents have employed. Parent guidance can be less effective when parents are not acknowledged as the experts on their child early on, for example, because the therapist may try previously used unsuccessful strategies. Parents may also feel unheard and undervalued. When therapists do acknowledge and listen to the parents' unique expertise with their child, future interventions can be co-created with all of the shared information.

STRATEGY: *Collaborative Expertise*

Though we are all under pressure to intervene quickly, remember to start every new treatment with both partnering and a thorough assessment, recognizing the significance of our partnership with the parent to create a foundation for change. You may have ideas early on in the process about how to intervene, based on your expert training and previous experience, but remember to "slow down" and allow the caregiver to tell their "whole story" about parenting the child in question. Sometimes, taking a deep breath and remembering that each family is unique can help. Let the parent know that you "get" the importance of their knowledge about their child, and appreciate the critical partnership that will be necessary in order to create change. You could say, for example, "Though I am a psychologist, I don't have all of the information necessary to help your child. You are the expert on your child. You are in the position to carry out suggestions and observe the changes in your child. The suggestions I make have to be a good fit for your child and for you. I am determined to work together as a team so that you and your child can feel better."

STRATEGY: *Convey Confidence and Knowledge without Arrogance*

You want to acknowledge that, whether you are a parent or not, the caregiver has more expertise and experience with their own child than you do. Be mindful of using language that families do not understand or of talking down to parents. Either one will let them know that you are not understanding where they are and what they bring to the table. Just stepping into the professional setting, a huge and desperate step for some parents, or having you, the professional, meet with them, will be enough to set the stage for some parents. Others will be looking for additional cues to your expertise: for these parents it is helpful to explicitly let them know about your experience, either about your general training or experience with a specific presenting problem. If you don't have experience with their presenting problem, be honest. Expressing your interest in learning goes a long way. Do not worry if you are in the early stage of your therapy training or career. You can still transmit confidence, even though you won't be able to say, "I have decades of experience treating this particular problem." In these instances, your supervisor will be guiding your work, and their experience will be brought to bear on how you move forward.

Sharing your professional experience with a presenting problem or situation is one way to inspire confidence and develop a healthy alliance in parent guidance. For example, if a parent asks if you have ever seen a child who behaves the way their child does, responding that you have worked with many children with similar behaviors, or have a supervisor who has, will convey confidence and hope.

STRATEGY: *Don't Overwhelm the Parents*

Some parent guidance sessions are rich with many observations and recommendations. The discussion moves quickly and fluidly. When that happens, summarize the suggestions and focus on one or a few things to try in the following week. Consider the following example. Once JDS and a pediatrician were providing feedback and recommendations to parents following a multidisciplinary evaluation. The pediatrician went through the findings and mentioned a bunch of next steps. The child had developmental delays and needed many interventions, including occupational therapy for both fine motor skills and sensory concerns, speech and language therapy for delayed speech, behavioral interventions for managing challenging oppositional behavior, and educational support. The parents looked like the proverbial deer in the headlights. JDS, noticing the looks on their faces, said, "So there are two basic things to focus on" and recommended interventions that would be used at school and behavioral interventions to help them manage at home. She then explained how the other items mentioned fit within those two categories. The parents visibly relaxed and then were able to talk about what to prioritize and what would be the concrete next steps.

One session might cover many topics. Perhaps you discussed bedtime routines, mealtimes, and homework. Several ideas arose for each.

> THERAPIST: We've talked about a bunch of different things today. It's a lot to remember, let alone try, in 1 week. What feels like either your highest priority or the one you are ready to tackle?
>
> PARENT: If we could get bedtime to go more smoothly, I could relax for a little in the evening. That would be great!
>
> THERAPIST: Okay. So we talked about creating a bedtime routine and also about working on Isabelle's trouble in falling asleep on her own. Let's go over the specific ideas and think about how to implement them.

Here the therapist summarizes, narrows, and hones in. Next the therapist will get specific and troubleshoot with the parent. The therapist does not suggest working on everything they talked about in that session, with the thought that a lot will get better at once. Rather the therapist recognizes that that would be a setup for failure.

Self-Disclosure

In the context of child therapy and parent guidance, the parent will ask some predictable questions, especially related to your credentials and parenting status. Before answering, you can query how this information will impact the work you are doing together. Be mindful of the tone you use, as this should not serve as an awkward or discordant moment, but rather a way to examine why this is important to them. If you choose to provide any self-disclosure, keep it focused on what will benefit the client. Sometimes self-disclosure can assist in improving the partnership by making the relationship feel authentic. However, the therapist must always remain focused on the goal: the parent guidance work. Otherwise base your decision about self-disclosure on your comfort level, your theoretical orientation, and what you think will be most therapeutic.

Two examples of self-disclosure may be illustrative. In one example, EB's father had died while she was at work. She did not choose to share this information with her patients. However, she had a department secretary who canceled her appointments for her. While doing so, the kindly secretary told EB's patients that her father had died, rather than saying something vague. Unfortunately, when EB returned to work, her clients asked many questions about his death, such as how he had died, how old he was, and how was she doing. One client even stated, "How can I ask you for help with my minor problems when I know you have something much more major going on?" This disclosure shifted the focus of the therapeutic relationship, and EB had to work hard to get therapy back on track with a few clients. In this case, the information was detrimental to the therapy.

Contrast this with a much more thoughtful disclosure. A female clinician, who happened to be married to a woman, was working with a child and consulting with the parents, who were a lesbian couple. The parents did not seem comfortable with the clinician and often had an irritable edge when interacting with her. The clinician brought this concern to her supervisor, who suggested that the parents could be assuming that the clinician was heterosexual and that she was therefore uncomfortable, judgmental, or homophobic. The supervisor suggested that the clinician, only if she felt comfortable doing so, make some comment to let the family know that she was in a same-sex relationship. The clinician chose to do so, with only one comment and no further discussion. This completely changed the tenor of her relationship with these parents, and it allowed the therapeutic consultation to continue in a much more productive way.

Figure 2.2 provides a guide to help you think through self-disclosure.

Some clinicians choose to disclose particular information about themselves, such as parental status, because they feel it is important in the therapeutic process. Considering the following questions can help ensure the process is thoughtfully done.

- What about me do I feel is important to disclose in doing parent guidance?
- Why would it help a caregiver with whom I work?
- When is self-disclosure a benefit?
- When is too much self-disclosure a problem? What are the potential or foreseeable problems?
- How do I know if there is too much self-disclosure?
  - Is it taking up too much time in session?
  - Is my patient starting to worry about me or asking me about things in my life?
  - Am I getting into casual conversations that are not in the service of developing the patient's comfort?

FIGURE 2.2. A careful look at self-disclosure.

CHAPTER 3

An Assessment to Guide Treatment

In parent guidance, assessment provides the information needed to formulate an understanding of the child's and caregiver's needs in order to determine the best course of action. Mash and Hunsley (2007) explicitly state that "there is a general consensus regarding the need for the development of assessment strategies not as an endpoint, but as a prerequisite for planning, implementing, and evaluating effective and efficient services for children" (p. 4). We focus on the elements that are critical for an initial assessment in parent guidance.

JDS worked with a supervisor who asked her after each assessment interview, "Did you ask about X?" He would then comment that he always asked about "X." "X" was always something different that she was "always" supposed to ask about. Finally, in exasperation, she asked, "How do you always ask about all of these things?" She and her supervisor laughed. She was left with the understanding that there is always more you could ask about, even when being thorough. We are not expecting that clinicians will always ask every question, but instead be mindful of what kinds of things to ask about and why. In considering your template for parent guidance assessment, there are many avenues to explore that cannot all be addressed in an initial assessment. Just as the "partnering" continues through the treatment, so does the "assessment." Think about the need to shift from the mindset of a finite assessment product to an ongoing process that includes an early formulation.

When doing parent guidance work, we must assess the interaction between the parent and child, individual factors within the parent and the child, and the bigger environmental factors, including the whole family, that may play a role in both the genesis and maintenance of the problem. Though the child may be the explicit target for change, the assessment may reveal the many outside forces, including the parent response, impacting the child's life and functioning.

Assessment of Attachment and the Parent–Child Relationship

PACT: "A" for "Assess"

Unique to parent guidance is the need to better understand the relationship between the parent and child and to recognize how that relationship plays into the clinical picture before us. After repeated similar interactions with a caregiver, both parent and child develop a rhythm and a way of interacting. Discern typical interaction patterns between the caregiver and child. The quality of the early attachment style has been correlated with multiple behavioral and relational outcomes later in life (Sroufe et al., 2005).

Unlike child therapy assessments, in a parent guidance assessment, it is beneficial to find out about the parent's attachment not only to their own child, but also to both their own parents and their imagined child, who existed before the child was born (Brandon et al., 2009). Fraiberg and colleagues (1975), in an influential article in the field of attachment, discuss all of the previous generations of parents (including grandparents and great-grandparents) or "ghosts in the nursery" and their unsettling—particularly in the case of maltreatment—and continued presence in, and impact on, the life of the current dyad. Knowing about the traumas, errors, and the ways of interacting of the previous generations is important for understanding how the parent you are working with currently views parenting. It may also be useful to find out about the more positively named "angels in the nursery" (Lieberman et al., 2005), or those family members who would have conferred a beneficial parental impact.

Figure 3.1 lists areas and factors to consider when thinking about attachment.

Learn about the Parents' Early Family Relationships and Attachment History

The caregivers' relationship with their own parents is likely to reveal much about their view of parenting. General questions such as, "What were you like as a child, and "how would your parents have managed this?" can begin the conversation. What caregivers learned from their own parents may also emerge naturally in sessions. The comment "If I did that with my mom, I would have been . . . " gives you information about their attachment history.

When taking a family history, include information about the parents' upbringing. What were the parents' family constellations? What kinds of parenting strategies did their parents employ? What are their feelings about that upbringing now? What does this information tell you about the attachment between the parent and the child? What were the hazards they faced growing up, both from their parents and from the wider community? Did the parents' caregivers protect them? Children are more at risk from emotional hazards when their parents are, because of their own difficulties, unable to buffer their children (see, for example, Goodman & Brand, 2009; Somers, 2007; Sturge-Apple et al., 2006). Possible questions to ask caregivers include:

- "What were your parents like?"
- "Were you similar as a child?"
- "Is there anyone in the family that was similar to your child at their age?"
- "What did you learn about parenting from your parents?"
- "What do you do the same way?"
- "Is there anything different about how you parent?"

Effective Communication

- How do the child and caregiver communicate?
- Are there warm and connected moments?
- Does the caregiver respond to the child's messages?
- Are there confused messages (saying one thing but meaning another)?
- Does the caregiver soothe the child when distressed?
- Does the child let the caregiver know about feelings and events in their life?
- Does the child use the caregiver as a "secure base" to explore the world, coming back for help when things go wrong?
- Does the caregiver provide support when the child is afraid, sad, or mad?

Boundaries

- Does the caregiver act as a supportive adult as opposed to a peer?
- Does the caregiver respect the child's boundaries?
- Does the caregiver rely on the child for emotional support more than is appropriate?

Confidence in Parenting

- Does the caregiver appear clear about the role of a parent?
- Does the caregiver appear "present" when with the child?
- Does the caregiver appear afraid of the child?

Quality of Touch and Tone

- Does the caregiver touch the child gently?
- Does the caregiver portray a general sense of positivity toward the child?
- Does the caregiver respect the property of the child?
- Does the caregiver denigrate or make fun of the child?

Attention

- Does the caregiver attend to the child's words and play?
- Does the caregiver maintain proximity with the child?
- Does the caregiver spend time with the child?

Concerns?

- Does the caregiver do anything that concerns you about their relationship with the child?

FIGURE 3.1. Attachment considerations in the parent–child relationship.

For example, one mother struggled to validate and provide positive feedback to her child. She worked on it in parent guidance, telling her therapist that she was validating her child, as the therapist had recommended. One day the mother and child were in the waiting room before the child's therapy appointment. The parent guidance therapist observed the mother tell her child, "I hear what you are saying," and then quickly followed with "but that does not make any sense because . . ." When the therapist brought this up, the mother revealed that she did not know how to "validate" her child because her own parents disputed her feelings when she expressed them. Given her own experiences with her family, she required more direct instruction on how to speak with her child about feelings.

Hear the Parenting Story

It is valuable to understand the story that led to this person becoming a parent. Did they always wish to be a parent? How did the reality of parenting match their fantasy about it? There is a convincing body of research (Cataudella et al., 2016) that even before babies are born parents develop ideas about who they are and start on the attachment journey. Your questions about parenting should start before the baby was born but also should include the pregnancy and birth, or adoption, finding themselves parenting when they did not expect to, such as in some kinship foster placement. The differing narratives of unplanned pregnancies, pregnancies that result from the years and money spent on fertility treatments, or pregnancies that work smoothly with everything going according to plan are very different narratives. These parents may all do well, but their journeys are unique and worth attending to, as this information impacts how you partner with them and intervene. One way to get to the parenting story is to give parents Worksheet 3.1, "Sentence Completion for Parents."

In one example, a family consisting of a mother, father, and child were seeking an evaluation of attention-deficit/hyperactivity disorder (ADHD) for their child. When asked about prenatal history, the mother whispered to the provider that the child was adopted. She whispered the information because the child ostensibly did not know, although the child had suspicions. It was a kinship adoption, meaning that the child was adopted by biological family members. It became clear, during the assessment, that the secret about the adoption, their worry about the behavior of the biological mother, and related separation anxiety were much bigger problems than the possibility of ADHD. The treatment focus shifted from assessment and management of ADHD to parent guidance targeting the revelation of the family secret.

Other Important Strategies in Assessment

Gather the Family Psychosocial History

The family psychosocial history, which includes each parent's background and social context, is also important. Understanding the family culture will help you align interventions with that culture, rather than creating a mismatch in the process. An awareness of the intergenerational factors, such as trauma and alcohol use, will also allow you to target your approach more effectively.

Within that context, learn about how the family identifies ethnically and culturally. Your interpretation of parental behavior, for example, may vary, depending on racial, ethnic, or cultural identity. Responses to parent behavior and interventions targeting parenting, should also take this information into account. For example, Dearing (2004) points out that restrictiveness on the part of Latinx and African American parents in poor neighborhoods is protective for the children.

Also find out about whether the family identifies with any religion, whether they practice their faith, and whether they find it a source of support, as many families do.

Understand the Parent–Child Dyad

Turning to the family in treatment, consider the parents' demeanor and feelings toward the children in the family. Do they enjoy being parents? Was the child a cuddly baby? Was the child easier or harder at a different age? If there is more than one parent, be cognizant of each parent's attachment style, views on parenting, experiences in their families of origin, and connection to each other. Watch for and ask about how they parent as a team. Do they enjoy any activities and time with the child? How do they imagine the child feels about them?

There are other relational clues. What does the parent know about the child's interests? If the child is interested in Pokémon, does the parent know what that is, the names of any of the characters, or how Pokémon evolve? The caregiver need not own their own Pokémon cards, download Pokémon GO, or watch the television show. It is more important that they can engage with their child and express that their child's interests are worthy of attention. When you find out what kinds of activities caregivers enjoy doing with their child and how they perceive the child's strengths, you will get a sense of the relationship. Asking about discipline or how they manage challenging situations will also clue you into the connection between the parent and child.

Observe Parent–Child Interactions

If parent guidance is part of the child therapy, you will have an opportunity to observe how the family interacts. Given the opportunity, observe all of the caregivers interacting with the child, with other children in the family, and with each other. If you are doing parent guidance without working with the child, ask about their interactions in detail.

In your observation, attend to both verbal and nonverbal communications. Do they sit near each other? Do they appear comfortable with each other? What are the apparent emotions? Is there overt or covert anger or resentment? Does the caregiver answer for the child or allow the child to respond for themself? If they disagree, how do they resolve their disagreements? Do they use friendly joking to lighten interactions. or do they use unpleasant sarcasm to undercut each other? These interactions provide cues regarding the quality of the attachment, the ongoing relationship between the child and the caregiver, and how effectively they resolve conflict.

Part of the observation, or inquiry if only parent guidance is involved, should be to assess whether the parent–child interactions are developmentally appropriate for the child. It can be a tricky for parents to adjust as their children grow, providing a push toward independence while also providing sufficient support.

Individual Child and Parent Factors to Assess

In order to complete a parent guidance assessment, you must understand the parent, the context, and the whole child in question. The presenting problem will be impacted by factors within both the parent and the child.

Temperament

Parents and children come into the world with different temperaments. Temperament is seen as emotional reactivity and excitability (Kandler et al., 2013) and has been shown to be relatively stable over time (Kopala-Sibley et al., 2018). Chess and Thomas (1984) wrote about different temperamental styles, including easy, difficult, and slow to warm. Importantly, one aspect of parenting work is helping the caregiver understand both their own and their child's temperament in order to gain a better understanding of how to interact in the most productive ways.

Evaluate the Match between the Caregiver Style and the Child's Needs

Identify whether there is a match or a mismatch between the parents' style and the child's style. Although many caregivers expect that their child will change to suit their preferences, we have found that expectation to be unrealistic. Some questions you can ask about the child's temperament include:

- Are they easygoing or reactive?
- Do they need downtime, or do they prefer to zip from one activity to another?
- Are they high energy?
- When they are upset, do they retreat or do they get in the caregiver's face?
- Are they very serious, or do they use humor effectively?

Use similar questions when asking about the parent's temperament. Talking about the match between what the child needs and the caregivers' style is a positive way to remove blame from the adult while still suggesting that they make some changes. One way to clarify temperament may be to discuss the different temperaments of the family members, which is especially helpful if they have children who present differently. For example, they may have one child who is easygoing and would float through life no matter what parenting style they were presented with, and another child who has a more difficult temperament and who would benefit from adults around them responding in certain ways. Be careful that this discussion does not lead parents to believe that you are recommending that one child's temperament should rule the roost. Rather it means that it is no one's fault that one child needs more help to improve their emotional and behavioral regulation than another.

Also get a sense of how well the parents work together. The parent can tell you if they feel that they are successful and effective in managing their child's daily routine and in deescalating their behavioral outbursts. They will likely be able to let you know if one parent handles these issues more easily than the other.

Assess How the Caregiver Understands the Child's Developmental Level

Parents often have an inadequate understanding of their child's developmental level, expecting more mature behavior and emotional understanding than children are capable of. When thinking about the child's developmental level, remember to query about psychosocial, cognitive, emotional, and physical development. Developmental level may not be consistent across domains. Further, there may be finer-grained variations in developmental level, such as a child who has weak visual-spatial skills and much stronger verbal skills, a pattern that often deceives parents about their children's emotional abilities, because the child's utterances sound highly mature, while other aspects of functioning appear immature. Inconsistent development across domains can be difficult for a child and confusing for the adults around them. An understanding of their child's developmental level will lead to appropriately targeted interventions.

Understanding the Parent's Personality, Strengths, and Pathology

Therapeutic work with parents entails an understanding of adult personality and pathology. In order to be successful as a parent guidance provider, an assessment of parental pathology and diagnoses is as important as understanding and assessing the child's difficulties. Ask the parent about their own mental health history and speak with their therapist if they have one and allow it. Though you are not looking to be both an individual therapist and parent guidance consultant, you will benefit from an understanding of the parent's medical and mental health needs.

Understand the Parents

Ask about the parent's diagnoses, mental health struggles, and psychotherapy. Common signs of parental difficulties include disruptions of sleep, eating, or thought; hyperactive behavior; difficulty following a train of thought; unusual thinking; and consistent negative or low mood. What stressors (home, work, parenting, family of origin, etc.) are they trying to manage? An awareness of these concerns in the assessment phase allows you to both target interventions effectively and also maintain a nonjudgmental and supportive stance. For example, during a parent guidance assessment, a mother shared that at the time of her child's first birthday she had been undergoing treatment for cancer and was not able to hold the child on her lap to eat her birthday cake. This mother's current treatment struggle involved eating issues for the child, who was now 7 years old. Having the information about the mother's cancer treatment and her concerns dating back to that first birthday, including her own feelings about herself as a mother, the therapist was better able to understand why feeding became such a unique focus. Going forward, the mother was able to address issues around food much more confidently, and the child's behavioral problems around eating became a nonissue.

If mental health concerns become a centerpiece of your parent evaluation, think about referring the parent to individual therapy. Some caregivers are also more aware than others are of their own foibles or behaviors that contribute to the parenting difficulties. Even though such self-awareness can be useful, it may also be a hurdle to overcome if their self-focus leads to judgment and blame rather than attention to making a change in parenting. People with mental health concerns are by no means excluded from parenting. It is extremely rare that a person's symptoms would be severe enough to preclude them from becoming a parent. Most caregivers with psychiatric issues are able to do a fine job of parenting. A strong protective attachment can form within the context of, or despite, significant pathology.

Don't Forget Strengths

Do not forget to ask about strengths. When parents struggle with their own mental health concerns, it is especially important to ask about their strengths, because you can build on them. Knowing their strengths will also help you appreciate the parent as a multidimensional individual with something to bring to the table in this work.

It is not just about asking the caregiver to say something nice about themselves or their child. In an assessment, it is important to be aware of not only what the parent talks about, but also what they leave out. Do they share any positives about themselves or their child? It says something about the relationship if the parent overfocuses either on the child's problems or the child's strengths. This information attained early on in the assessment phase helps not just in understanding the situation, but also in setting the groundwork for you and the parent to capitalize on in the treatment phase.

Strengths may include a value that the family shares, a propensity to being logical and linear, being "psychologically minded," or loving the child despite not knowing how to improve the situation, to name a few. If your focus is on strengths, you are likely to have success early on that will build hope and stamina for engaging in the process. For example, if the caregiver is very organized, developing a tracking tool for behavior may feel very productive to them. These strengths will help you in multiple ways, including developing your own empathy for the caregiver, achieving early success, affording opportunities to praise the caregiver, and identifying qualities or areas around which to build interventions.

Assessment Beyond the Individuals and the Relationship: Other Relevant Data

Understanding Concerns and Barriers to Care

After gaining a basic understanding of the individual caregiver factors, the next phase of the assessment will be to understand the environmental concerns in the life of the family and the barriers to effectively accessing care. Some caregivers may be able to jump right in with whatever you suggest. Others may have more barriers, including skepticism, that may make it difficult.

Think about the Goals

Part of the assessment involves gaining a clear understanding of what the parent hopes that the therapy will change. Can the parent articulate goals? How will they know if the situation improved? What does better look like? It may be that the parent prioritizes something very different from what the parent guidance clinician would prioritize. For example, in a case involving their child's severe sleep disruption and suicidal gestures, one parent was most concerned about the child's grades.

Explore a Day in the Life

Though you will not observe it directly, you can still learn about the family's daily routine. What does the family's day look like, from the time they wake up through the nighttime routine? Asking about a typical day cues the parent to provide information that they may not recognize as important. How do the members function together? Where are the trouble spots in a typical day? Do the parents and child, or children, spend enjoyable time together?

Investigate Barriers to Parent Guidance

Assess the reasons that parents may have trouble accessing care. Think about Maslow's (1943) hierarchy of motivational needs, considering that when more basic needs are not being met, it is extraordinarily challenging to work on higher-level needs, including self-improvement or self-actualization. Some of these barriers may include financial factors, job insecurity, food and housing instability, or medical concerns in the family. Other barriers, including a lack of time and transportation, may involve problem solving, such as, for example, getting Medicaid insurance to cover transportation, and being realistic about what is reasonable to expect from the parents.

Another possibility could be that the family did not feel welcome or represented when they showed up in your waiting room. Or perhaps their neighbor saw someone for therapy and that person (reportedly) said the most outlandish thing, and as a result the family does not trust therapists. Maybe the child's pediatrician suggested they seek therapy, so they are coming to you not because they want to, but because they feel that they have to. Ask about their thoughts and feelings about therapy, including about parent guidance. Worksheet 3.2, "Gaps and Needs to Figure Out in My Parenting Life," found at the end of the chapter, can help caregivers concretize what could be helpful for them.

Collect Data

Consider asking the parent to collect data about a specific behavior between these early assessment sessions. Although this is not done with all parents, gathering data can clarify the frequency and pattern of the concerning behavior and provide a baseline from which to assess whether your intervention strategy is producing change. In the context of recording data, parents become more self-aware of their own behavior and can often be more consistent in their responses.

Needs, Difficulties, and Strengths: The Road between Assessment and Choosing Your Intervention

With a thorough assessment, you as the therapist have a lot of puzzle pieces to put together. Think about your formulation and your understanding of the parent, the child, and the situation, recognizing that it will evolve as you continue working with this family. Communicate your formulation, including the parent's needs and appropriate strategies, with the parent. Remember that your understanding of the caregiver's skills and needs will play into not only what you tell them, but how you do so.

Clearly the presenting problem should impact the intervention you choose. Does the parent's story of the problem fit with your formulation? You think that the child's anxiety is the fundamental issue, but the parents think it is their oppositional behavior. Do you work on oppositional behavior, or do you provide psychoeducation to the family to help them understand why you think that the anxiety is leading to the oppositionality? How do identified strengths change your plan? Do they signify which interventions will be most effective or how you will deliver them? This early formulation is the next step to choosing effective strategies, setting you up for the next stages of treatment.

CASE STUDY: Understanding Caregiver Barriers

A kinship foster mother was referred for parent guidance work, as she was having difficulty implementing changes that would be helpful for her foster daughter. Significant trauma therapy had to be done with the child, but a critical piece of that work involved the foster parents. However, only the foster mother brought the child in for most sessions, and she struggled to be more emotionally available for this child and had a hard time understanding the child's needs. While she was well intentioned, the foster mother was not open to working on changing her own style when responding to the child.

The clinician thought carefully about her formulation. The factors to consider included the history of trauma, the child's signs and symptoms, the child's openness to therapy, the stability and longevity of the placement, what the foster mother was capable of or willing to do, and the involvement of the foster father. The child had experienced trauma and was demonstrating trauma-related signs and symptoms. Although she was now in foster care in a safe home, she lived with a caregiver who was not willing to engage in active therapeutic work to support her. Knowing this, the clinician made calculated decisions about what to focus on in the session the foster mother. Because the foster mother was willing to meet with the therapist to talk about the child's behavior, the therapist met her where she was, recognizing the limitations in her ability to display more empathy for the child. Instead, they worked on very concrete strategies that met the requirements of what the foster mother felt were important, such as around respectful behavior, while also creating a more nurturing environment for the child.

This chapter described many factors that need to be considered in a parent guidance assessment. Figure 3.2 summarizes prompts that you can use.

After partnering and completing the formal assessment phase, the next step is choosing and implementing the most appropriate interventions, as discussed in Part II.

Parent's attachment history:

- What were you like as a child?
- What was your upbringing like?
- What was your relationship like with your parents?
- How did your parents manage emotional and behavioral challenges with you?

What is the parenting story?

- How did this child come to be in this family?
- What were your expectations of parenting?
- If this is a biological child, how did you feel during the pregnancy? What was the birth like?
- Was it an easy or difficult pregnancy?
- If this is not your biological child, how did they come to be part of your family?
- Do you have information about the biological parents?

Parent's family background and social context:

- Cultural identification
- Ethnic identification
- Religious identification
- Socioeconomic experiences

Relationship with the identified child:

- Describe your relationship, both in the past and now.
- Do you enjoy being a parent to this child?
- What are your child's strengths and interests?
- What do you enjoy doing together?
- What is your child's temperament like?
- What is your temperament like?
- What do you expect of a child of this age?
- What supports do you have?
- What stressors are you coping with, including any ongoing medical issues?
- What are you struggling with (including mental health concerns)?
- Are you involved in your own psychotherapy?
- What are your family routines?
- How is behavior management handled in the home?
- What goes well in the family?
- What are your strengths and interests?

FIGURE 3.2. Prompts for a parent guidance assessment.

WORKSHEET 3.1

Sentence Completion for Parents

The most important thing about being a parent is ______________________________

____

I feel effective when ____

____

The best thing about being a parent _____________________________________

____

The worst thing about being a parent ____________________________________

____

Children rarely ____

____

My favorite thing my child does ____

____

My favorite game when I was a child _____________________________________

____

Children often ____

____

A moment I enjoy most days is ____

____

A moment I struggle with most days is ___________________________________

____

As a parent I am really good at ____

____

Something I look back on and laugh about is ______________________________

____

Three qualities I want my child(ren) to have are

1. ____
2. ____
3. ____

WORKSHEET 3.2

Gaps and Needs to Figure Out in My Parenting Life

Emotional

Example: Someone to vent to

Example: Someone to bounce ideas off of

____

____

____

____

____

Concrete

Example: After school pickup

Example: Getting the roof repaired

____

____

____

____

____

Day-to-Day

Example: Homework help

Example: Making chores happen

____

____

____

____

____

PART II

What You Need to Know to Choose Effective Parent Guidance and Develop Parenting Skills

This part of the book focuses on the times when parent guidance would be an effective intervention strategy and when it would not be. Launching parent guidance requires a thoughtful and intentional decision-making process. These chapters help you to avoid the common error of jumping in with a strategy, such as a behavior chart, before identifying the best ways and times to intervene. Here we also discuss developing and reinforcing fundamental parenting skills, which are useful in general but particularly when children have emotional and behavioral challenges.

CHAPTER 4

Developing the Path for Intervention

PACT: "CT" for "Choose" and "Treat"

After partnering with the caregiver, and learning more about the family and their situation, it is time to choose an intervention path and begin treatment. How do you choose the best course of treatment, matching the intervention to the reason for referral as well as to situational, parental, and child elements? How do you make the decision with the caregivers about what to do next? The following detailed list offers the factors to consider in the delivery of parent guidance as your treatment modality.

1. *Is the problem likely to improve with parent guidance?* If the parent has the power to make the problem better, then parent guidance can be a very helpful endeavor. Parent coaching is useful when the parent is making the problem worse through lack of skill, their own emotional dysregulation, a lack of understanding of their child's behavior, or a lack of ideas for managing complex situations. When the problem is outside of the caregiver's control, it will likely yield less-than-stellar results. Some situations in which parent guidance is unlikely to help include those in which parents are frequently arguing, in which they cannot commit to treatment, or in which a whole-family intervention would be more helpful.

2. *What skills does this caregiver have that would aid or impede parent guidance?* In the assessment, consider the parent's ability to be self-aware and reflect on both their own feelings and behavior as well as the child's. What is the caregiver's current repertoire of parenting skills and their ability to change? Are they interested in adding new skills, and are they able to?

3. *What resources does this caregiver have that would aid or impede parent guidance?* The resources that families need to successfully participate in parent guidance include:

   a. *Time.* The caregiver needs to be able to take time away from work or parenting other children to be able to attend. They need to have the time to carry out the suggested interventions, which likely includes spending time with the child.
   b. *Energy.* They have to have enough energy to engage differently with their

child. The identified child patient is likely not the only drain on their energy. While they may understand that over time interactions with their child will take less energy if the work is successful, they still need to implement what you agree upon. Instill hope, and a vision of change, to help them muster the energy.

c. *Money.* The parent needs to have the financial stability to pay for the appointments. Some families struggle to manage a copay much less a full-fee session with a parent guidance expert. If part of the parent guidance interventions involves reinforcers and attending fun activities, consider what the family can afford before recommending them.

4. *What values does the caregiver have that would aid or impede an intervention?* Are they open to parent intervention? Some parents believe that the children should be the ones to change and perceive interventions directed at their behavior as offensive. Does the parent believe that parent guidance would be helpful both to themselves and their children?

5. *Acuity of the problem:* Most often the concerns that present in your outpatient office are appropriate for that setting. There are times when a child or parent needs a higher level of care than can be provided by solely utilizing outpatient psychotherapy. An emergency room evaluation is a good place to start when the parent or child is not safe. If the child is at risk but does not need the emergency care offered in a hospital, you can help them consider the following options: residential care, in-home family teams, day treatment, and specialized schools. These programs provide more hours of care to address entrenched problems that cannot be tackled through parent guidance and child therapy alone. However, parent guidance is a useful adjunct when outpatient therapy is suitable for the parent and their child is involved in a higher level of care.

6. *Would the parent benefit more from their own individual, couple, or family therapy than from parent guidance?* We assume, in parent guidance work, that parents and other caregivers play a critical role in the behavior, emotional functioning, and development of their children. An obstacle to helping their own children can be the mental health concerns of the caregivers themselves. Caregivers of children with behavioral problems have higher rates of depression than the general population, although they are unlikely to receive direct therapy for it (Gopalan et al., 2011). Acri and Hoagwood (2015) highlight the importance of intervening to address parents' needs when children suffer from mental health concerns.

There are some situations in which parents participate in both individual psychotherapy and parent guidance work. The individual therapy provides enough support so they can benefit from the parent guidance work. With greater attention to their own mental health, the caregiver may be better able to implement interventions that would assist the child.

Other signs that an individual or couples therapy referral would be warranted include significant conflict between the parents and an inability to keep the sessions focused on helping the child. When the caregivers disagree about more than the management of the child's needs, couples therapy about the bigger conflicts can be more helpful than parent guidance. Though it may be uncomfortable to suggest psychotherapy for the adult, do so if the parent's mental health is a barrier to helping their child. Broach the subject in the context of offering more support for the caregiver.

If it would be useful to bring the whole family, or the parenting unit, together into the change process, family therapy may be the best choice. Consider referring to family therapy when you notice the following: one of the children is always identified as having difficulties, but a different child is identified each time; communication is generally difficult; the family is not working as a team; family members "feed off each other" in negative ways or feel misunderstood; or family interactions are a significant source of the difficulty.

7. *Are you the right match for this caregiver?* Maybe the parent would work more effectively with a provider who is similar to them with regard to demographics, such as age, gender, or race. Respecting the caregiver's wishes about who may be the best fit is an important part of the process.

8. *Do you have the skills needed to help this caregiver?* Sometimes a specific psychological intervention requires skills that you do not have. For example, maybe a parent wishes to help their teen manage cutting behavior, and you think that helping the parent learn the basic tenets of dialectical behavior therapy (DBT) would be beneficial in helping that child cope and progress in their own treatment. Do you have the training to do this or should you refer the caregiver to someone who does? Despite the fact that there may be techniques that you have not been trained in, you do not always have to refer out at the first sign of something slightly new to you. Assess whether it is something you can learn through training and consultation, or whether the intervention required is such that you need to refer out.

9. *Would the child benefit from another adjunctive service?* No single therapy, including parent guidance, solves every family's problems. In helping the parents we work with, we must know when and how to refer and collaborate with other professionals, outside the realm of psychotherapy, to find the best program for each struggling child. Parents do not always know about or know how to access these services.

Imagine these scenarios:

- *A family is referred to you because the child does not follow instructions.* You develop a sophisticated rewards and consequences program to improve listening skills, only to discover that the child has a hearing loss or a language-processing disorder.
- *A family is referred to you because their usually happy child is suddenly lethargic and is having difficulty getting up for school.* You believe that this is depression and begin to help the family alter the child's thinking, only to find out that the child's signs and symptoms are thyroid related.
- *A family seeks your help because their child is not applying themself in school.* You work with the family to set up an organized workspace and to encourage parental support for completing homework, only to later learn that the child has a specific learning disorder.

All of these initial interventions seem reasonable. However, they unfortunately lack an understanding of the reasons for the behavior and, therefore, are not solving the problem at hand. The reasons for the behaviors, in these scenarios, can be ascertained by referring to other professionals. See Appendix B for a more detailed discussion of services that families can be referred to.

When to Intervene

The Benjamin Franklin quote "An ounce of prevention is worth a pound of cure" should be the motto of parenting. No one ever regrets preventing a problem, though they may never know what disasters were averted. Parents typically enter treatment with their children when a problem already exists. We must remediate the problems presented to us, though no remedy can compare to never having had the problem in the first place. In parent guidance, our larger goal going forward is to help parents recognize their contributions to problems, identify what they can do to be more helpful and effective, and create new patterns and strategies that reduce difficult behavior, emotional distress, and mental health problems in their children.

Why do so many parents resist engaging in preventive parenting? Some parents believe that their children *should* behave differently than they do and that parents should not have to scaffold, predict, and prepare the environment for success. As therapists, we believe in prevention and attempt to understand the barriers parents have to using it. Parents may underestimate the value of having a positive, nurturing, and collaborative relationship with their child. Other parents have said that using prevention strategies takes too much time, neglecting the obvious—how much energy and time it takes to argue with a child or deal with tantrums. Sometimes parents believe that children will be made "dependent" and will not learn the skills they need to manage their emotions on their own if they are assisted in dealing with dysregulation.

Pregame, Game, Postgame

We have identified three potential intervention points to help parents deal with difficult child situations. Using the analogy of a sporting event can help parents recognize potential points for them to intervene with their child. They include vulnerability points and opportunities prior to the difficult behavior, during the challenging behavior, and after the behavior has occurred. Your recommended strategy will be different, depending on when the parents decide to intervene.

1. Intervene before anything goes awry. This is the "pregame," or the time before the difficult behavior occurs when caregivers might recognize a problem brewing and intercede in order to avoid it. Just as a coach knows their team's strengths and weaknesses and makes a game plan based on them, a parent can recognize what situations are likely to be problematic for their child and can plan accordingly. It involves the foundational skills and parenting practices that either prevent issues from ever occurring or minimize their impact. We consider the pregame time the most effective point

at which to intervene. You may find it difficult to convince parents to intervene before there is a problem because the challenging child behavior may be the primary catalyst for action, or they may have difficulty identifying key moments before there is a problem. Even though usually parents attend therapy when there is an established problem, you can determine the proactive strategies that will help improve the behavior that brings them to you and use them early in treatment. Similar strategies can also be useful later in treatment when you may be "fine-tuning" family functioning.

2. The midst of a struggle or difficult situation with the child, which we call the *game*, offers your next potential point of intervention. Similar to during a sporting event, strategies during the game can be reactive rather than contemplative. This is often the most challenging, and yet most often tried, time in which parents intervene. Despite its lack of effectiveness in creating lasting change, parenting energy often goes to the game, because when behavior that is dangerous, destructive, or hurtful is happening, it cannot be ignored. Though we prefer proactive pregame interventions, we can and often do help caregivers understand more effective ways to manage at the game point.

3. After the situation has passed, there may be a quiet time to learn from events, build new skills, or create a different outcome in the future. We call this time the *postgame*. During the postgame we can help the parent reflect, with the child or on their own, on events and emotions in order to develop healthier solutions. The postgame is often a time when all parties are motivated to change. Beware that sometimes "after-the-fact" behaviors, such as apologies and expressions of regret, can sustain the negative behaviors by repeatedly allowing for the child to fix, or repair, the situation. While behavioral repairs can be useful, when the same behavior happens time after time and the repairs do not appear to change it, it is worth trying a different tack. Thinking carefully through the postgame helps determine a plan to alter the negative behavior, which may, ironically, sometimes include eliminating these reinforcing (wiping the slate clean) niceties.

How do these different points of intervention play out? Here is an example in which the same issue is managed at all three intervention points. Imagine that a child, who has previously had tantrums at birthday parties, is invited to one. The problem is predictable, as it has occurred before, and a plan can be made. The parents tell you about the birthday party pattern, which you explore in greater depth. You ask essential questions, such as when does the tantrum start, what are the triggers, what does the child say when they are distressed and after they have calmed down, and how does the situation end. In this example, the parents tell you that their child functions well at parties until the gifts are opened, but at that point the child tantrums (cries and kicks adults) until the child is "dragged away" from the party. Calming occurs when the child is back home and having a snack or playing quietly.

Pregame

Your first step in the pregame is to help the parents recognize the pattern and then proactively make decisions about how to manage it when it occurs in the future. At this stage of intervention, parents can make environmental changes, such as skipping the party, if they believe the child will not be successful. They can also remain at the party to supervise, if appropriate. They can choose to pick the child up before presents are opened, since this time is predictably when their child melts down. But better than any of these avoidant strategies would be a plan to help the parents work with the child to manage the situation more effectively. The parents can write a social story about parties that includes coping strategies. With your help, they can alert the child to predictable feelings, behaviors, and strategies to manage their feelings. The parent can practice, with the child, the strategies you identify, such as rehearsing scripted comments (i.e., "It will be my birthday soon") or going to another space when presents are opened. If these feelings and behavioral options are previewed, it may be easier for both the parent and child to recognize when the child is feeling distressed but has not yet lost control. Caregivers can also preemptively script deescalation strategies for themselves, including their own comments to have ready in response to both their child and bystanders, recognizing that these moments are stressful for everyone.

Game

During the game, the parents utilize the strategies they identified in the pregame as the party is underway. If they did not utilize pregame strategies, the intervention starts at the game. There are many reasons why parents may not have utilized the pregame interventions: maybe they were not aware of the birthday party pattern, they may not have had the time or inclination to address it before the event, they may wish that the problem did not exist, or they may have exhausted their repertoire of interventions and not know what to do. Suppose the scenario plays out, and the child is dysregulated and crying. The parents must respond in the moment to the child's behavior, which may involve removal from the party, trying to calm or restrain the child, and/or do damage control, with both peers and parents observing the situation. During the game, anything that exits the family from the situation or returns the child to baseline functioning may feel like a win. Yet there may be unintended consequences for overreliance on this intervention point, such as reinforcing and practicing negative behavior, avoidance of the difficult situation if exiting is the solution, building a community narrative that the child is difficult, bolstering the child's belief that it is very unfair when other children get presents, or the child developing ingrained negative thoughts about themself such as "I cry all the time." The essential problem in starting the intervention at the game point is that no matter how masterful the response to child behavior, the undesirable behavior still has the opportunity to happen.

Postgame

Athletes and coaches review what did and did not work in the game plan in order to improve performance in the future. Similarly, parents and children both benefit from processing after the fact in order to gain a better understanding of their own triggers and to develop strategies for future use. Was the problem predictable? Should the parents utilize the same pregame interventions, if they had any, or fine-tune them next time? What happened and why? Self-awareness can be developed for both parent and child: "Parties are supposed to be fun but you seem sad when you're there"; "You have trouble controlling your body when other kids get presents." These moments of self-awareness can then be linked to planning for the future and reducing distortions.

The postgame can also be used when the child did well, and the child and parent can reflect on strategies that they used to cope: "I think we had a good plan about the party" (reviewing the specific parts that seemed to work). The postgame can also involve practicing skills, such as saying, "Thank you for inviting me" (social etiquette) or "It will be my birthday in a month" (self-soothing) or "Parties are fun even when you don't get presents" (reducing distortions). Thinking about the timing of the intervention with the parents helps them generate solutions to build a greater sense of control.

Use Worksheet 4.1, "Identifying the 'Game,' " to help caregivers review key ideas and moments in the pregame, game, and postgame approach.

WORKSHEET 4.1

Identifying the "Game"

How do I know we are in the pregame? How can I intervene now?

What is happening, about to happen, or likely to happen?	What patterns do I recognize?	What has worked before?	What skills do I want to develop?	What tools do I have in my toolbox?	Let the games begin!

How do I know we are in the game?
What can I do to get through it?

Uh-oh, here we go!	What can shorten this episode?	How can we all get through this?	Is everything safe?	What tools do I have?	Phew, it's ending.

How do I know we are in the postgame?
What can I do now to make this moment better and improve things in the future?

Is my child really calm enough to process what happened?	What lessons can I take from this moment?	What lessons can my child learn from this moment? What skills can my child develop?	How can we communicate about this moment productively?	How can we move on from this moment?	Maybe next time things will be a little better.

CHAPTER 5

Strengthening Optimal Parenting

The prevention toolbox is predicated on the idea that effective parenting can reduce child mental health and behavioral concerns. As a mental health provider, you can help parents develop the skills and strategies that lead to better outcomes by circumventing some problems altogether and reducing others when they arise rather than inflaming them. Most of the strategies we present for teaching parents can be incorporated within a variety of therapeutic styles and treatment plans.

Optimal parenting assumes that there are strategies for caregivers to employ that promote family well-being. As a parent guidance expert, you should have ideas about best parenting practices even in the absence of mental health concerns. What makes a strikingly good parent? How can you tell? Do they set firm and clear limits, while conveying warmth? Do they encourage independence, while providing needed support? Are they able to read their child's cues well and respond in helpful ways? The strategies provided in this chapter serve to prevent problems as well as recognize areas in which caregiving can improve.

Creating Nurturing Moments

Imagine the success we would have as parent guidance experts if we were able to increase the number and quality of nurturing moments between children and their parents! Research shows that nurturing environments play an essential role in the prevention of child mental health concerns (Biglan et al., 2012; Sroufe et al., 2005). When mothers were more responsive and comforting to their crying infants their babies cried less over time (Ainsworth et al., 1978). This finding is in direct contrast to the behavioral expectation that by responding to crying, and therefore reinforcing it, crying would increase. We see nurturing as a need similar to the needs for sleep and food, rather than something children earn or manipulate parents to get. Creating an environment in which children can signal their needs and explore their environments within the context of support and availability is an important recommendation to deliver to caregivers (Sroufe et al., 2005).

In order to encourage moments of connection, we should be able to describe what a nurturing environment is and help parents begin to create it with their children. Can they tenderly hold their child? Can they look at them with love? Do they share moments of joy? These optimal nurturing moments build trust and collaboration as an everyday part of the parent–child relationship. You can utilize the following list of concrete recommendations to develop and enhance nurturing moments.

1. Identify times when the parent is most available to connect with their child.

2. Review the bedtime routine to determine whether moments of connection, such as reading together, cuddling, singing bedtime songs, or having meaningful conversations for older children can be added. Alfie Kohn (2005) pointed out that a frequent penalty for young children who have misbehaved is taking away their nighttime reading and cuddling with parents. He sees this decision as a missed opportunity for "righting the boat." Children are often worried about the relational rupture that their misbehavior causes, and this bedtime provides a unique postgame moment that sometimes parents are too angry to avail themselves of.

3. Help the parents identify interests the child has that they can explore together.

4. Help caregivers figure out if there are ways children can help, such as in preparing family meals. Can the child stir what is in the mixing bowl? If the child is too young to truly help, can they cut up their toy food while the parent cuts up the real food? Also help parents set reasonable expectations for the quality of the help; it's okay if the child will likely not cut evenly or not stir thoroughly.

5. Determine a place in the home that can be used as (or redesigned to be) a place for nurturing. Goodyear-Brown (2021) has many structured suggestions on how to create a "nurture nook" for families. Designating a spot with a beanbag chair, stuffed animals, books, or pictures and posters is a good start. Of course, this is not the only place where such nurturing moments can take place but, for some families, having that spot designated encourages them to happen.

6. Figure out shows, movies, or audiobooks that families can enjoy together. These activities are not only enjoyable in and of themselves, but also lend themselves to physical connection, particularly with younger children.

7. Developing shared interests and activities, like a mutual hobby, can provide new topics for positive discussion and moments of connection.

Child-Led Play/Teen-Led Activities

Despite spending a lot of time together, some parents may not typically play with their children. There are clear benefits to parent–child play for skills development, social-emotional functioning, and improving family relationships (Yogman et al., 2018). Parent–child play is also strongly recommended by many parenting programs that target difficult child behavior. There are different names for it, ranging from "special time," "child-led play," and "child-directed play," but there is sound agreement about its role in improving parent–child relationships and increased adherence to family rules (Barkley, 2013; Eyberg & Bussing, 2011; Greenspan & Wieder, 2006; Kazdin, 2008; Webster-Stratton & Reid, 2010). Child-led or child-directed play is a specific kind of play that is seen as improving family communication because parents follow the child's lead, rather than telling them what to do, as they often do in daily life.

In child-led play, parents often experience an epiphany about how directive driven they are. They also recognize how hard it is to not take the opportunity to teach, especially if there are aggressive themes or cheating to correct. Remind the parent that these issues can be addressed at other playtimes that will occur in the future. Give them the language to use in challenging situations, such as saying, with a playful tone "You really like to win. You are using your own rules." Teach parents the skill of reflecting, or simply narrating, what the child says or does. When children lead, they rarely choose the "educational" options that make parents feel that the time is being used in a valuable way.

Note that this intervention can be applied to teenagers as well. We both did child-led play/teen-led activities with our own children. One of us (JDS) played Super Smash Bros. with her teenager because it was of interest to him, although she would not play video games on her own. And one of us (EB), map in hand, repetitively searched around her home with her child looking for every orphan in France, resisting (most) urges to change it up.

In introducing child-led play, many parents will need instruction about how to let the child lead. Parents often wish to suggest what to play, picking a more palatable choice for themselves. You can help by suggesting that they practice the following:

- Reflecting statements ("You like that block").
- Neutral questions ("What is your baby's name?").
- Mirroring statements (reiterating something the child has said).
- Asking, rather than telling or suggesting ("How do you want to use our time together?"; "Okay, I'm the doctor. What does the doctor do?").

There are other challenges beyond those involved in the difficulty of following a child's lead. Help parents figure out how to handle them, because engaging in child-led play does not come naturally in many families:

1. Troubleshoot with the caregivers. This may involve thinking through their schedule and determining when child-led play will fit in. They may need to figure out how to focus on one child at a time when there are multiple children in the household.
2. Siblings can be competitive about whose "special time" it is. Encourage parents to plan ahead, which can reduce sibling competition if there are multiple children at home.

3. Make sure that parents understand what it means to follow a child's lead. The adult should not correct or teach. They should not change course unless indicated by the child. Unless there is a safety issue, they should let the child direct.
4. Caregivers can reflect what they see, noting what the child is doing. Demonstrate with parents, and have them practice in session if reflection is difficult for them. Modeling clay or drawings are quick-and-easy vehicles through which they can practice reflection. The observer can reflect the actions, affect, and words of the person using the modeling clay or doing the drawing. Phrases such as "You are using a lot of green in that picture," or "You are hitting that clay really hard!" demonstrate reflection.
5. If the child casts them in a role, the caregiver can ask the child what they are to do in that role.
6. Remind caregivers that it is okay to be playful and that they may enjoy the experience.

If several weeks go by and the parents have not engaged in this activity, try to figure out what the barriers may be. Sometimes there are time constraints. Parents may not be comfortable playing or allowing the child to lead. You can try to reduce the barriers, but if a parent is still reluctant, do not judge. In this case, try to focus on other interventions. Though child-led play has some specific advantages, encouraging any play between parents and children is beneficial.

Building Parents' Skills in Conversing with Their Child

Many parents and children do not communicate well with each other. Communication problems may be why there have been multiple reprints over many years of *How to Talk So Kids Will Listen & Listen So Kids Will Talk* (Faber & Mazlish, 2012) and *Between Parent and Child* (Ginott, 1969) that instruct parents on this topic. Part of your role in providing parent guidance is to help parents figure out how to have productive conversations with each of their children.

In everyday life the role of parents can involve directing the child with a series of commands ("Time to go," "Get your shoes," "Brush your teeth"). Developing listening opportunities and communication skills are important and can help the parent get to know about the child's interests, friends, and concerns

Conversation Suggestions

Though parents often want to talk at the dinner table, these conversations can become one-way streets focused on parental opportunities to plan, issue commands about desired behaviors ("Did you tell your teacher about the missing assignment?"), or inquire about school. Some conversation starters can be more invitations than demands, however, and may be more productive. Suggestions to stimulate more open conversations include the following.

- Have rituals, such as asking about the "rose and thorn" of everyone's day.
- Talk when not facing each other directly, such as when driving in the car, doing a task like cooking, walking, engaging in a sport, or playing games together.
- Show interest if the child has a passion (such as cosmetics, popular music, or construction toys).
- Reduce sarcasm. Sometimes parents communicate with their children in unhelpful ways. Sarcasm, distinct from humor, is rarely if ever a useful way for an adult to engage with a child.
- Eliminate insults or slights. Notice in their recounting of family events whether parents also provide compliments that function more as insults, as in "caboosing" (Kazdin, 2008), or saying something nice but adding a comment that ruins the compliment, such as "You cleaned your room well for once," or "You did what I asked. That's a shock." Parents are often unaware that they are speaking this way, and self-awareness can decrease this pattern.

Teaching Caregivers to Look for Repetitive Themes

When speaking more with their children, parents discover that the children often focus on repetitive themes. As repetitive talk can become boring to the adult speaker, it is tempting to dismiss children's immature interests and questions. Ginott (2003) believes that when children ask the same question repeatedly there is meaning that is worth exploring. Ironically, parents feel dismissed when they receive no meaningful answers to questions such as, "How was school?" but similarly sometimes do not want to discuss the child's juvenile interests. If children bring up a serious topic, provide space for them to talk about it and have their concerns and questions heard. If a topic, such as death, surfaces repeatedly, it is probably not coincidental and bears further examination. In summary:

- Teach caregivers to listen to their children, including attending to themes.
- Script language that will be an invitation for the child to talk more, such as "You are concerned about X." Reflection in this instance can be used to good effect.
- Help parents tolerate conversations about difficult topics, such as death, sexuality, and drug use.

Communicating an Understanding of Feelings

Many caregivers can benefit from learning how to let their children know they "hear" them and can handle their distress. What do we do when we do not feel heard? We get louder (until and unless we shut down). When children do not feel that their parents "get" them, they may escalate their signals to get their message across, which can take the form of literally yelling louder or engaging in increasingly difficult behavior. Clinicians can help parents do the following when their children are distressed:

- Tolerate that distress.
- Reflect back what they understand.
- Talk about the concerns with their children.
- Validate the child's feelings.

These skills allow for open discussion and encourage addressing emotions, problem solving, and language skills. The conversations develop a vocabulary of emotions, a tolerance of challenging feelings, and the development of a coping repertoire. Concrete strategies caregivers can use to demonstrate an understanding of feelings include:

- Reflection, which involves reflecting back what the child is saying or doing or how the child seems to be feeling (If the child says, "I am sad," the parent can say, "I see you are sad").
- Active listening, to show that the listener is really attending (eye contact, leaning in, nodding).
- Behavioral description ("I see that you are playing with Play-Doh now").
- Asking questions (about what the child is saying or doing). Differentiate this strategy from "grilling" the child about topics they would prefer not to talk about.
- Making comments that indicate joining without judging or evaluating ("I can see why you would feel sad about that").

When we teach a parent to communicate that they understand where the child is coming from, they can help reduce the affect and then pave the way for intervening in more helpful ways.

The Importance of Routines and Rituals

Maintaining Regular Routines with Flexibility

Many children function well with predictable routines, such as those provided in school. A frequently postulated rationale for why children behave better in school than at home is the clarity of expectations and consistency of schedules: Children know what to expect and what is expected of them. An important healthy habit to encourage parents to practice is the development and maintenance of a positive daily routine (Fiese et al., 2002). A routine involves completing things that need to be done, such as getting dressed or brushing teeth, in a predictably patterned way. Some keys to creating routines include:

- Identify the times of day when regular routines would be especially helpful, including getting ready in the morning, coming home from school, preparing for dinner, and going to bed.

- For younger children, a pictorial representation of what is expected and in what order makes the routine work more effectively. Older children and adults can use checklists if needed.
- Bedtime may be the most important time to develop a routine, as the transition to sleep is challenging for many children. Though some rituals may seem inconsequential to adults ("I love you to the moon and back" or a special number of kisses), they provide tremendous reassurance to children. If bedtime is handled successfully, it provides the reward for parents of either time to accomplish tasks or to pursue their own interests and relationships aside from the children.
- Though some kids need the routine to be more inviolate than others do, almost all children rely on predictability.
- Before a routine is established, help the parent make certain it is doable for everyone, including the parents and siblings.

Worksheet 5.1, "Smooth Routines," can help caregivers think through how the routines around their regular activities are going and how they would like them be better.

Building in Rituals

Rituals as used here imply a meaningful and intentional way of marking events such as births, deaths, holidays, and graduations. They do not always center around a major event or holiday. Rituals can be powerful individualized ways to center the person and the relationship. For example, there was an extended period of time when one of us (JDS) would come home from school without her siblings. She and her mother would have a cup of tea, two cookies each, and a discussion about the day. Though it was unplanned at first, it became meaningful. Rituals, in both daily life and for bigger events, help anchor us and give a sense of direction. Some families have weekly family movie nights or pizza Fridays. Rituals do not have to develop organically, nor do they have to be handed down from generation to generation. When there is a big change, such as a death or divorce in a family, there is an opportunity to develop new rituals. You can facilitate a discussion around creating rituals:

- Help caregivers identify rituals that they already engage in as well as how various family members enjoy and gain from them.
- Consider the holidays that are important to the family. For example, on Halloween the child may benefit from knowing there will be pumpkin carving. Children may require less novelty than adults.
- If there has been a marked change in the family system, help the caregivers identify or create new rituals.
- Find smaller events that can be ritualized, if that would be useful to the family. This could be a special breakfast together on a weekend morning, a special greeting in the morning, or a particular after-school snack and chat.

Parent–Child Activities That Promote Good Mental Health

Exercise

Do the family members, including both parents and children, exercise? Building in regular exercise has positive effects on mental health (Rodriguez-Ayllon et al., 2019). Helping parents and children move a little each day is likely to improve mood, attention, and anxiety. In fact, a study (Bowling et al., 2017) found that the small introduction of twice-weekly cycling improved kids' behavior and classroom performance.

Relaxation

Relaxation has recently been shown to be effective in reducing anxiety (Alvarez et al., 2015), consistent with older research finding improvement in anxiety, stress, and mood dysregulation (Platania-Solazzo et al., 1992). Though less formal means of relaxing, such as listening to music and watching television, can be valuable, distinguishing these informal versus formal relaxation strategies may be advisable. You can encourage parents to incorporate daily *formal* relaxation programs for themselves and their children to reduce the overall level of stress at home. In the "olden days," we would have made a relaxation audio cassette with a personalized script for the child to use or taught parents to make a tape with our help. Currently, professionally produced relaxation programs abound, and there are also a host of online scripts available if you want to return to the old-fashioned way of doing it (see Appendix A for resources). If families are open to the idea, incorporate a relaxation program into your parent guidance practice. Since families have different preferences for ways to relax, you can offer them progressive muscle relaxation, breathing techniques, body scans, basic biofeedback, and guided imagery, to name some.

Mindfulness exercises also help many people become more relaxed. In our experience, there are people who benefit more from active mindfulness exercises, such as walking, and games that require one to pay close attention, rather than the more traditionally "relaxing" ones. One example of a more active mindfulness activity is the "Snap, Crackle, Pop" game, during which people stand in a circle and need to pay attention to the word said (snap, crackle, or pop) and the associated arm movement. Another fun mindfulness activity can be trying to balance a feather on one's open hand. Experiment to see what works for the particular person in front of you. Although teaching each of these exercises is beyond the scope of this book, it is important to remember that the parent and child's interests, skills, and values may play a role in which of them you select to use.

Not all of the strategies listed in Figure 5.1 involve traditional relaxation techniques, but they do help children relax or reregulate their mood. Some are particularly helpful when children have trouble engaging in more typical or formal relaxation activities.

- Create a coping box with them.
- Have a place where they can blow bubbles.
- Learn several breathing exercises that you can practice with them.
- Have music on hand that they enjoy and find fun or relaxing, and that makes them happy.
- Create a cozy nook (beanbags, pillows, stuffed animals, pictures, books).
- Read together.
- Give them space (even if they slam the door).
- Be silly with them.
- Take them outside for a walk.
- Suggest a shower or bath.
- Let them talk about what is bothering them without trying to solve the problem and without getting upset.

FIGURE 5.1. How parents can help their children reset their mood.

Parent Self-Care

Caregivers may not always be able to improve their child's level of happiness but they can engage in self-care to improve their own. Parent self-care is something that is always recommended but may be hard for some parents to follow. Many parents cringe at the word "self-care," suggesting that we should perhaps choose a new name for this activity. Choate (2016) convinces mothers to help themselves, both for their own sake and also for how doing so models self-care for their daughters. In creating a self-care plan, remember that what seems beneficial to one person may be stressful for another. Self-care can only work if it is reasonable to do in the timeframe allotted and does not create more stress on the other end, factoring in what was not accomplished.

- Encourage parents to recognize that self-care activities can be in-the-moment, in the short-to-medium term, and in the long term (Kinniburgh, 2014). For example, it may be helpful if a parent recognizes that they are becoming dysregulated in the moment to close their eyes and imagine feeling a cool breeze in a forest, to sing a few lines of a particular song to themselves, to repeat a parenting mantra, or to smile a little. In the short-to-medium term. these quick strategies for self-care may help them get through the moment and then they can do something more to make themselves feel better and more regulated. This could include reading a book they enjoy or having a cup of tea. Long-term self-care might have to do with exercise routines, eating well, or planning for retirement.
- Have caregivers create a list of what helps them feel better and address barriers to engaging in those activities.
- Identify ways that parents can bring additional moments of joy into their lives.
- Review pleasant activities lists and Worksheet 5.2, "Relaxation for Parents," to help stimulate ideas.

Strategies for Building Hope and Goal Setting for Caregivers

Develop a Vision of Where the Family Wants to Wind Up at the End of Treatment

Heath and Heath (2010) suggest creating a destination postcard with caregivers. The idea of a destination postcard is that you cannot make things better if you have no concept of what better would be. Efforts to increase awareness of both the problem and what "better" would look like make it easier to approach the change in small steps. Helping parents identify goals may start with thinking about how they wished parenting would be, how it truly is, and ways to bridge that gap. The "miracle question"—asking, "If you woke up tomorrow and a miracle happened so that you no longer had ____ problem, what would you see differently and what would the first signs be that the miracle occurred?" (De Shazer et al., 2021)—is another tool that can be used to help the caregiver imagine what "better" would look like.

Goals That Are Focal and Build toward a Target

Once you identify the "destination" or goal, it is useful to set specific steps that work toward that objective. Breaking down problems and generating small steps toward solutions recognizes that change happens gradually, and is more similar to turning a dial than flipping an "on–off" switch. The following scenario is an example.

THERAPIST: So your goal is for your child to get through a whole weekend in a good mood with no tantrums?

PARENT: Yes, that would be amazing!

THERAPIST: It will be! Let's figure out some steps on the way. It's not that we will hit on one solution that, all of a sudden, makes it so Lorelai has no distress for a full 2 days. You have to work up to it. What is a time that is typically a little hard for her?

PARENT: Waking up on Sunday morning. We go to church, and she doesn't mind Sunday school, but she is a bear to get out of bed and that sets the tone for half the day.

THERAPIST: So let's start with that. We'll work hard on making that time of day go more smoothly and then expand from there. What do you think?

PARENT: That would make a big difference.

THERAPIST: Let's not assume that we'll come up with some way that gets her to open her eyes with a big smile on her face and hop enthusiastically out of bed. What would be a more reasonable first goal?

PARENT: Me waking her up and her not yelling at me.

THERAPIST: All right. Let's start with that.

Create Family Mottoes and Belief Systems

Goal setting can be more of an exercise in figuring out what values and practices suit the caregivers' family. In the book *The Secrets of Happy Families,* Feiler (2013) outlines powerful tools, such as developing family stories and traditions, which foster collaboration among family members. It can be rewarding for a family to allow you to help them create a positive family story. These stories can be the arrow pointing the family in the direction of growth. You can use Worksheets 5.3, "Our Family Story: Part I," and 5.4, "Our Family Story: Part II," with parents as a framework.

Convening the Family to Create a Compact

After identifying the "destination" and setting a path toward reaching it, families can create more formal agreements about changes for members to make. Family agreements are tools that can address disagreements or lack of clarity around expectations in a household. Bringing family members together to create a plan increases understanding and buy-in. Using a "Family Agreement," such as the one in Worksheet 5.5, may assist families in developing a plan.

WORKSHEET 5.1

Smooth Routines

Daily routine (i.e., meals, snacks, bedtime, getting ready for school, tooth brushing) 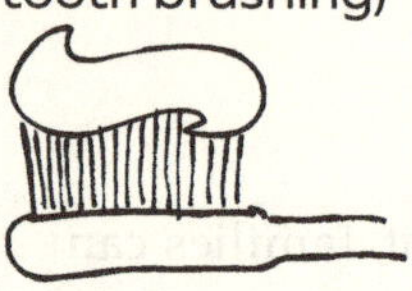	How does it actually go? 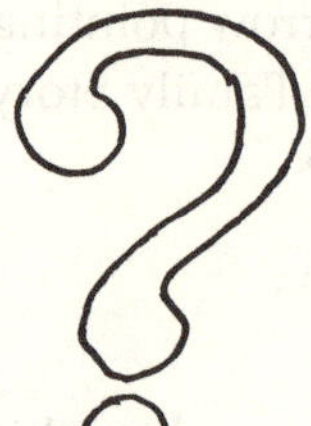	Stuck points 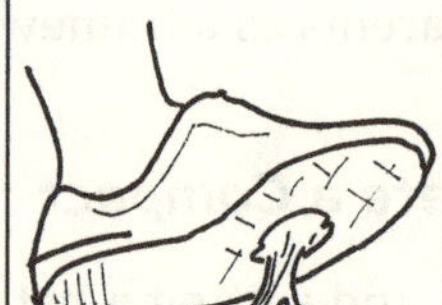	What would you like it to look like? (aspirationally) 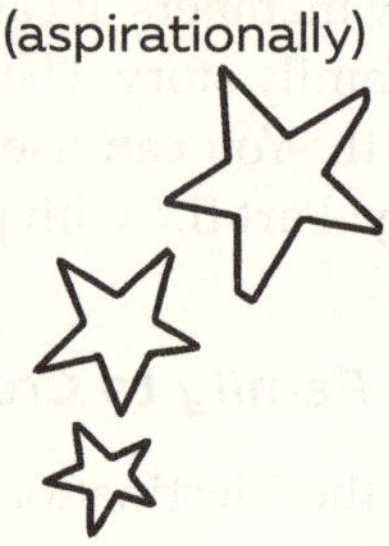	What might get you closer to that aspirational routine? 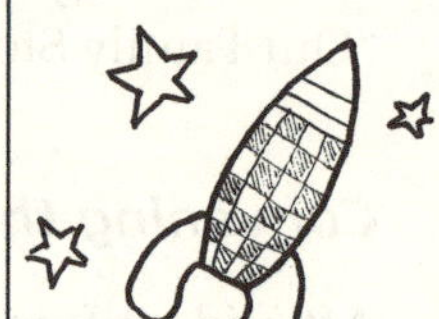

WORKSHEET 5.2

Relaxation for Parents

What helps relax me?

____ Breathing

____ Imagery

____ Reading

____ Audiobook

____ Calling a friend

____ Exercising

____ Music

____ Coloring/Drawing

____ Handcrafts

____ Being outside

What else?

Which relaxation techniques can I access easily? Can I make any others more accessible?

Do they really relax me? How do I know?

How often do I use my relaxation strategies? Do I use them enough?

WORKSHEET 5.3

Our Family Story: Part I

These prompts will help you develop your story.

Who is in my family:

1.
2.
3.
4.
5.
6.

How did we come to be a family?

___

___

___

What is wonderful about us?

___

___

___

What has been our journey?

___

___

___

Where are we now?

___

___

___

Where are we going? What is our wished-for epilogue?

___

___

___

WORKSHEET 5.4

Our Family Story: Part II

WORKSHEET 5.5

Family Agreement

We are coming together about ______________________________

____

____

It is really important that we ______________________________

____

____

We all agree to try

1. ______________________________
2. ______________________________
3. ______________________________
4. ______________________________
5. ______________________________

If it does not work, we will try ______________________________

____

____

____

____

We will not

1. ______________________________
2. ______________________________
3. ______________________________
4. ______________________________
5. ______________________________
6. ______________________________
7. ______________________________

CHAPTER 6

Building Proactive Competence in Parents

It is much easier to build consistent, healthy patterns than to remediate difficulties. Ideally, we work with caregivers to prevent emotional and behavioral problems in their children. There are many techniques that parents can learn and use effectively to help stave off challenges. This chapter focuses on ways parents can assist their children through skills building, planning, and organizing.

Building Parents' Awareness of Their Child's Behavior

Identify Skills the Child Is Missing and Teach Them

One of the main tenets of collaborative problem solving (Greene, 1998) is that "kids do well if they can." This runs counter to the theory that children behave poorly to get attention, and instead proposes that most people would choose to do well if they could. It helps parents to know that their child does not enjoy misbehaving. Rather they lack skills in frustration tolerance, emotion regulation, flexibility, and delay of gratification (Greene, 1998). Work with the parents to identify their child's lagging skills. It is a positive starting place for planning interventions, though it is likely not intuitive. You can increase caregivers' understanding of the child's behavior using these strategies:

1. Explain to caregivers the idea that children are lacking cognitive, emotional, or social skills. The concept that problems occur as a result of lagging skills, as opposed to intentional meanness, alone can make a difference in the caregiver's understanding of the situation, and therefore in how they respond to the child.
2. Help the caregiver identify the situations in which their child behaves in suboptimal ways. What skills would be needed in order for their child to do better?

3. Determine what method would be effective. Would explicit teaching make a difference? Practice and role playing? Scaffolding?
4. Work with the parent to develop a plan, with reasonable expectations. Incrementally build this skill, thus changing the behavior.

Worksheet 6.1, "I Can Help My Child Develop," provides a simple guide for identifying the goals and skills needed.

Recognize That Most Expectations Are Met

Even the most disobedient children do much of what they are instructed to do by their parents. When parents say their kids do zero percent of what they are asked, nonjudgmentally inquire whether they eat meals, go to sleep, or attend school. Recognizing compliance when it does occur is of value in altering parents' negative cognitions and feelings of hopelessness about their offspring. It also allows parents to look more specifically at their child's behavior, helping them to alter their own all-or-nothing thinking. The following dialogue provides an example.

PARENT: My child never does what I ask them to!

THERAPIST: Never? Most kids do some things that their parents ask, though it really can feel like they never do. The times when they don't do what we want really stand out. Can we talk about this a little and see if that is what is happening?

PARENT: Okay.

THERAPIST: So tell me a little bit about a typical day.

PARENT: Well, Kevin gets up at 6:00 A.M. to get ready for school. He showers and gets himself some cereal. I ask him whether he finished his homework, and he gets angry right away. He starts yelling at me, and when he leaves for the bus he says something snarky and slams the door. When he gets home, he goes right into his room and ignores me if he can. He comes out for dinner but eats as fast as he can and then goes back into his room. I don't know what he is doing. I don't know if he is getting his homework done. At some point he brushes his teeth and goes back into his room.

THERAPIST: It's really hard when your kid doesn't talk to you, except to yell and be difficult. There were a few things in there that sounded okay. He gets himself up in the morning, and you don't have to wake him?

PARENT: Yes.

THERAPIST: He gets himself together and out the door on time for school?

PARENT: Yup. But he knows I won't drive him if he misses the bus because I have to go to work.

THERAPIST: And he brushes his teeth without being reminded. Okay. So there are some basic things that you don't have to remind him to do. That's helpful. I have worked with a lot of teens who don't brush their teeth or shower, and it becomes a big source of tension.

PARENT: I'm glad we don't have those problems!

THERAPIST: It's good to hear that there are some things he does without reminders and fights. I think we can build on that. I know those fights hold center stage, but it is good that he does some things without reminders and nagging.

PARENT: I guess that is true. It could be worse.

THERAPIST: I know it can be really hard to keep that in mind, and we'll work on it together.

Modeling Better Behavior

Strategies to Help Caregivers

Model Patience, Flexibility, and Appropriate Behavior

Ironically, parents sometimes engage in the very behaviors that they wish children would not engage in. Children model what their parents do, not what they say to do (Rushton, 1975). Caregivers need to recognize that they serve as a model for their children. This means demonstrating patience and flexibility, as they would want their child to, as well as not behaving in a way that they would not want to see in their child. JDS had a client for whom this was a significant problem. Getting the first grader to stop calling her mother a "cow," when everyone in the family called every female a cow when they were upset, was extremely difficult! It is amazing how many parents wish their children would not curse when they themselves model this behavior. Identify those behaviors that the parent would like to use or would like to remove from their repertoire (changing problematic parental behavior is covered in Parts V and VI).

Use Self-Talk as a Tool for Children to Learn

When parents speak out loud, with their children within earshot, they model healthy thinking for their children, buy time, and coach themselves to remain patient. For example, when a parent and child see an ice cream truck, the parent can muse out loud, "I'd like to say 'yes' to the ice cream truck but we haven't had dinner yet, and I wonder how that will go. I am also wondering if I say 'yes,' if you will want ice cream whenever we see an ice cream truck." Overt and out-loud decision-making processes, such as balancing pros and cons, are a healthy way to improve children's flexible thinking.

The key in the use of self-talk is that it has to be a positive message for the child to hear. If the parent's thinking tends to be more negative ("My mother would have hit me with a belt for that, and I am trying to parent differently"), self-talk is contraindicated.

Even positive statements indicating the depths of the parents' concerns ("I can handle this. It's so hard to be a good parent") might be unnerving for a child to hear. Self-talk aids parents if it clarifies their thinking, slows them down, and calms their affect. Plan with the parent and talk through whether particular statements will be helpful or not if stated out loud to, or around, the child.

Help Parents Remain the Parents

When dysregulated, some people have trouble remaining parental. When parents cede authority to the youth, or act immaturely themselves, it creates problems. Peerlike behaviors include threatening to cry, speaking in baby talk, fighting and insulting as a peer might, begging, wanting the child to be an adult partner, and competing as a peer. Developing adult behaviors and avoiding the childlike ones can create a sense of safety for both parent and child.

Using Prediction to Preview and Plan

Predicting Difficult Behavior

The same events in families can transpire daily and yet be a surprise each time they occur. When a parent says, "Put on your shoes" to their second grader, they expect compliance, even if it has rarely worked. Many parents will say something "came out of the blue" but upon further investigation, there is a predictable pattern. If the child demands a slushie every time they walk by a shop, do not be surprised by the next slushie demand. When you predict, you can prepare an intervention!

Previewing and Planning

Previewing, or telling children in advance what to expect, builds executive functioning skills and reduces distortions and misperceptions, which are often a source of child distress. For example, when kids are at school all day, they may be imagining what they will do when they come home: "I'll eat my candy; I'll watch my favorite show; I'll have a playdate." When the parent picks them up and says, "We're going to the dentist," this news requires a gear shift that might be understandably upsetting and provoke challenging behavior. If the parent told their child the day before and paired the information with coping strategies or ways to think about the dentist visit, the distress is markedly reduced. For younger kids use visual aids and pictures they can refer to in order to boost the effectiveness of previewing. Predicting feelings and reactions to situations for children has been shown to be beneficial in reducing negative behavior (Park et al., 2020). Anticipating how events will work out reduces difficulties and anxiety for both parents and children (Trad, 1992).

For example, when JDS worked as an aide in a public-school autistic program in the Bronx, New York, there was one child who would become very dysregulated when the teacher was going to be absent. If she knew she was taking a day off, we would say repeatedly the day before, "Tomorrow Susan is going to be ____________." And he would say, "Absent." And then we would say, "And you are not going to ____________," to which he would reply, "Yell." It worked. The next day he was prepared and better able to cope. To sum up:

1. Identify examples of when previewing would be helpful.
2. If caregivers struggle with the words, develop flexible scripts with them. For example, they might use this language:

   PARENT: Normally on Wednesdays you have piano lessons. Your piano teacher called and said she was sick, so tomorrow you will not have your lesson. You will have some extra time. I will remind you tonight before bed and then again tomorrow morning.

   CHILD: Is she okay?

   PARENT: She just has a little cold. I expect she will be fine, but she needs to rest tomorrow.

   CHILD: Okay.
3. Role play with the caregiver. Start by demonstrating, and then encourage the parent to practice the previewing skill.

Use Social Stories

Gray's social stories (2015) provide step-by-step guides to previewing everyday activities, such as going to the dentist and brushing teeth. Though the social stories were originally developed for children diagnosed with autism, they have become an enormous aid for previewing upcoming activities, feelings, and coping strategies. They may describe a previously frightening event, such as a fire drill, and provide psychoeducation about the nature of the event and how to cope with it.

Parents often ask questions with regard to the best timing for previewing future events. For example, when a child has an upcoming surgery, we recommend previewing the sequence of events for them. Typical hospital guidance suggests previewing 1 to 2 days ahead for a preschooler and a week ahead for an elementary school student. Teenagers can learn about their surgery with their parents, with the caveat that individuals, especially with learning challenges or anxiety, may need modification of these timeframes. As with many planned events, parents can preview how the child can manage a medical intervention, such as what they can bring with them to help with distraction.

Previewing can also be used for predictable events that may be difficult to handle, such as a teen party with drinking, a friend being mean, making a mistake, or getting lost. It also prepares the caregiver for these possibilities in the lives of their children.

Bridging

Bridging occurs when one activity leads into the next, as in the image of a bridge getting you where you need to go. It is useful when it is hard for a child to transition, particularly from a favored activity to another activity.

For example, if a child loves the park, it may be difficult to leave. The first step with bridging is previewing with time reminders, such as, "In 5 minutes we need to leave the park." When telling the child about the need to leave, you can bridge to the next activity. "We have to leave the park to get ice cream" is a likely easy bridge, as getting ice cream is probably a preferred activity. Having to leave the park to do a less-preferred activity is harder, though adding another step makes it more palatable: "We have to leave the park to do homework and after that we can play a game!" Even with nothing preferred to offer, previewing with time alerts is a useful skill for parents to learn.

Organizing Tasks, Time, and Spaces

Building Frameworks for Daily Life

Previewing relates to the bigger strategy of building frameworks to increase success, sometimes called *scaffolding*. Scaffolding, in this context, involves a more skilled individual helping a less skilled individual become successful in a particular area. You can visualize scaffolding as creating the foundation so that children can be successful. One strategy is breaking a task down into steps so that a larger undertaking can be completed as a series of smaller parts. It may involve assessing task difficulty and making it easier without doing the whole task for the child. Examples of breaking down tasks include laying out clothes for kids to wear, waking kids in the morning who are not ready for an alarm clock, having a dry-erase board with instructions, or placing dishes where kids can see them to set the table. Building these frameworks may involve previewing with visual and verbal reminders, task analysis of what the child can currently do, and providing the assistance needed to successfully complete activities.

Strategies to increase child effectiveness in task completion include:

- Helping parents think about the following questions: "What does this whole task require, and where can I put in supports if needed?"; "What part can my child do?"; "What would be the next step to build more independence?"
- Celebrating progress and encourage caregivers to do so.
- Striking a balance, meaning creating a hospitable environment that also has minor challenges in order to build a child's skills. Sometimes parents can take the idea of making tasks easier to an unhelpful degree, trying to prevent any frustrations or difficulties from ever occurring. These parents are ever-ready to solve any problem, taking no risks at all about tasks that they cannot control, and have numerous rewards at the ready. It is through mastering these minor challenges that children learn the important skill of frustration tolerance. Providing accommodations to children who do not need them runs the risk of preventing

growth rather than encouraging it. A parent-friendly book that espouses this point of view, with multiple examples, is *The Blessing of a Skinned Knee: Raising Self-Reliant Children* (Mogel, 2008).

Recognize the Problems Caused by Time Pressure

When families are heavily scheduled, there is ample opportunity for arguments, as they struggle to get out of the door for activities on time. As Leidy Klotz describes in the book *Subtract: The Untapped Science of Less* (2021), we often try to solve problems by adding something in, when perhaps the more helpful solution is to remove something. This is likely challenging, but it may be worth talking with caregivers about the possibility of reducing items in the schedule or tasks. What may feel necessary may not actually be. An easier recommendation is to estimate more time than is needed to accomplish everyday tasks. Everything is harder under time pressure. Getting up earlier, aiming to get places early, or reducing the number of expected tasks in a given time improves everyone's mood and the situational outcome. This is an intervention you can suggest to parents when they report that they are typically late, rushing, or stressed about getting places, or if they are often late to see you. Everyone's mood and flexibility are affected when they have no temporal buffer. The following example models a way to have this conversation with a parent.

PARENT: Mornings are really hard. Everyone is rushing. We barely get out of the door in time. I wind up yelling at Nora and she starts crying. That makes us even later. I drop them off late and get to work late. It's a lousy way to start my workday.

THERAPIST: Sounds pretty lousy. While we are working on Nora's ability to stay calm and manage how she is feeling, let's see if there are some practical ideas to make the morning go a little more smoothly. What are the tasks that need to happen in the morning?

PARENT: Well, I get the kids up, which takes a while. I really need to be getting breakfast ready, but instead I am bugging them to get out of bed. They need to get up, change into their clothes, eat breakfast, brush their teeth and hair, and get their backpacks together. Then they put their shoes and jacket on.

THERAPIST: And what are the things you need to do?

PARENT: I get their clothes out, get their breakfasts and lunches ready. I have to shower and get dressed, eat my own breakfast, brush my teeth, dry my hair, make sure the kids have everything they need for the day and I have what I need for my workday, and get us out the door.

THERAPIST: That's a lot. When do you get up?

PARENT: I get up at 6:30 A.M. and get the kids up at 6:45 A.M.

THERAPIST: Do you do any of the tasks the night before?

PARENT: Not really.

THERAPIST: Okay, I have a couple of ideas. The first one is not usually people's favorite, but I'll throw it out there anyway. What do you think about getting up 15 or 30 minutes earlier? You could either get stuff done with that time, or you could enjoy a quiet moment before you get the kids up. Have a cup of coffee or tea before things get hectic.

PARENT: I don't know. I really like my sleep! But the idea of a quiet moment is kind of nice. I get things done much more quickly when it is just me.

THERAPIST: I bet! A lot of prep could happen in 15 minutes before anyone else is up. The other possibility I am thinking about is that some things could be done the night before. They might even become part of the nighttime routine. With less time pressure the kids could even do more of these things. Could they pick out clothes for the next day? You could check and make sure they are reasonable outfits, but they could pick them out? Or could lunches and backpacks be prepared the night before?

PARENT: They might like to start picking out their own clothes. If they got their backpacks together the night before, that would save a lot of stress in the morning!

Think about Household Organization and Spaces

Creating an organized, workable space in which to live can be an effective prevention measure. Ask parents about their home space and how it is working for them. Have them think about the different feelings engendered in a chaotic versus an organized environment. Sometimes interventions that create a functional space, such as getting a desk for a child struggling with homework, can be preventive.

As part of organizing, think about object placement. Parents can create less attraction to items that intensify family conflict and more attraction to desirable choices. For example, parents might complain that their children use items inappropriately, such as throwing balls in the living room. Keeping basketballs in garages or backyards can reduce such behaviors. Similarly, advise caregivers against putting a television, or other electronic devices if it can be avoided, in a child's room because the child cannot be expected to resist the temptation to use the device. If you want to increase specific behaviors, item placement may also assist. Why not have healthy food items at a child's eye level in a cabinet or up front in the refrigerator (Montuclard, 2017)? Get an alarm clock for the child's bedroom, so that the cell phone is not the de facto alarm clock. Environment, spatial design, and organizational choices make an impact on child and family behavior:

- Talk through the family environment and how it works and does not work for their child.
- Figure out ways that the caregivers can reorganize environments to create a greater likelihood of positive mood and desirable behaviors for both caregivers and children.
- Figure out if the parent can access some help, such as a family member who can aid in organization or cleaning.

Worksheet 6.2, "Helpful Changes in Our Family's Physical Space," offers a framework for parents to use in thinking about organization in this context.

One Final Word on Prevention

Prevention poses the *It's a Wonderful Life* problem. In this movie gem, Jimmy Stewart plays George Bailey, an admirably decent man, whose random positive interactions have saved his entire town. At the start of the movie, we see George, a broken man, ready to take his own life as many of his hopes and dreams have not been realized. With movie magic, George is shown what his town would have been like if not for his preventive actions. Unlike George Bailey, we cannot see what problems good parenting practices avert in each family, though it is clear that prevention makes for many fewer difficulties. Clinicians can help families recognize and appreciate that a positive change in baseline behavior represents progress.

Part III will address common problems that families face and strategies to manage them.

WORKSHEET 6.1

I Can Help My Child Develop

My child and I are working on:

1. ______________________________

   ____

2. ______________________________

   ____

3. ______________________________

   ____

4. ______________________________

   ____

Skills to develop:

1. ______________________________

   ____

2. ______________________________

   ____

3. ______________________________

   ____

4. ______________________________

   ____

Goals:

1. ______________________________

   ____

2. ______________________________

   ____

3. ______________________________

   ____

4. ______________________________

   ____

How I will know things are different:

1. ______________________________

   ____

2. ______________________________

   ____

3. ______________________________

   ____

4. ______________________________

   ____

WORKSHEET 6.2

Helpful Changes in Our Family's Physical Space

Spaces I would like to add (like a place for my child to study, a space for my child to relax, a space for me to relax, a space for my child and me to snuggle):

1. ______________________________

2. ______________________________

Spaces I would like to change (like an area that could be useful but is too messy right now, or my child's room has gotten kind of dilapidated over time and needs a bit of a makeover so they can feel calm and happy in there):

1. ______________________________

2. ______________________________

How do I reduce the barriers to making this change happen?

1. ______________________________

2. ______________________________

3. ______________________________

PART III

Choosing and Using Treatment Strategies

Intervening with Common Problems

When caregivers share the specifics of their day-to-day struggles with their children, certain topics come up repeatedly in sessions. We have dubbed these predictable sources of family stress the "usual suspects." Be prepared to address these common problems with practical solutions in your work with parents. The usual suspects we review in this part of the book include:

- Homework
- Bedtime
- Eating
- Hygiene
- Digital media
- Going to school
- Music, sports, and other extracurricular practice
- Sibling conflict

CHAPTER 7

An Introduction to Assessing and Addressing Common Problems (the Usual Suspects)

PACT: "A" for "Assess"

How do you identify the usual suspects, the frequent and predictable difficulties that occur in everyday family life? In the same way that the police investigate crimes, you use your knowledge of behaviors and typical causes of problems. Then you look for clues in the specific circumstance. What is the problem? When does it occur?

When a parent reports a problem with their child, follow that lead as Sherlock Holmes would. In this detailed example of sibling conflict, we describe following the lead of a specific parental concern. In this example, you can see how we might formulate questions; gain a fuller picture of what happens; and identify behaviors, feelings, and context. Though we present many questions that could be asked, this inquiry is not meant to be a rapid-fire cross-examination of parents nor a rigid script. Be thoughtful about your questions, and monitor the parents' reactions in your continued dialogue.

Steps to Understanding the Usual-Suspect Problem in Parenting Session Dialogue

"She just can't stop hitting her brother and there's no reason for it. When will it ever stop? She's a hitter. She does it all the time." This example is used to highlight the steps in understanding a challenging behavior.

Step 1: Get specific. Questions should focus on the troubling behavior, mood, or situation. Details are important here. How is the behavior described? Ask the parent to give you specific information, including about frequency, timing, duration, and severity. Ask for their theory about why they think it is happening. It is very unlikely that the child hits "all the time" and that "there's no reason for it."

If you don't get a clear picture, ask for more specifics. Sample details to think about include whether she is punching, slapping, or hurting her brother in other ways, the force used, the frequency of hitting, and how seriously he has been hurt. Include whether she uses weapons or throws items and whether she hits only her brother. The trajectory, including when the behavior started and whether it has gotten better or worse and under what circumstances, can be helpful to know. Ask your questions conversationally, and prompt for more information with techniques such as reflection. Your comment could sound like "So she hits him in the afternoon when she is supposed to be doing homework . . . " and see whether the caregiver then elaborates.

Keep probing until you feel that you have a clear idea of what the problem entails. Many times, we think we see a problem clearly, but we are actually making assumptions about it rather than understanding it.

PARENT: It's only in our own home, but it can be anywhere in our house. It happens a few times a week. Her brother hasn't been seriously hurt, though he cries. She usually hits him once and then stomps off to lock herself in her room. She hits him on the arm usually. Once she threw a pillow in his direction but she hasn't thrown other objects. Her brother is the only person she hits. He's so sweet and doesn't deserve it.

Step 2: Ask the parent to describe a particular time when this behavior occurred. Explore it in depth. Gather data. Get a detailed "before, during, and after." Sometimes when answering questions, parents become surprised by the obvious patterns they had not previously recognized. Look at the events that led up to the problem behavior as a chain with many links to understand better how each link leads to the next. In each step you will often have to prompt for more information. Sample prompts include the following: What did you see happen? Did something specific trigger it? What was happening for each of you beforehand?

THERAPIST: What happened?

PARENT: It was after school. She was playing on her iPad, taking a break from homework. He came home from school after she did. I heard him say "It's my turn." And why shouldn't he have a turn! She had been playing for a while. I heard a scuffle, and then I heard him crying.

THERAPIST: So you didn't see the interaction happen directly?

PARENT: No. But they both grab the iPad from each other all the time. We have one for them to share. They both get a half hour with it every day after school.

You might think we have sufficient information here, but we don't! How does the family measure that half hour of iPad time? When is it expected to happen? How should the siblings transfer the iPad between them based on the family rules?

THERAPIST: What was her mood and behavior before he came home?

PARENT: When she came home, she had clearly had a hard day. She barely said anything to me.

Step 3: Figure out the circumstances and environmental factors that made this behavior more likely to happen. Why did it happen at that time and place? Does it generally happen at the same time every day? Parents often say "It's random," but when you ask them to keep a record, they discover patterns.

THERAPIST: I wonder if she was hungry or tired. Maybe it was a hard day at school or there's something else going on in her life?

PARENT: She usually has a snack right away. I have it ready for her. She wouldn't tell me what happened at school, but Wednesdays are usually hard because she sees the reading specialist, who she doesn't like.

THERAPIST: What happened when your son came home?

PARENT: When he comes home, he's excited to play with her, and she just hits him.

THERAPIST: Wait a minute. Maybe I'm missing something. Did he want to play with her or use the iPad? What were his mood and his day like?

PARENT: Let me think about it . . . I think he is excited for his iPad time, and he's been in school all day. He's not great about waiting his turn, so he grabbed it like he often does. Then I heard him crying and assumed she hit him. When I ran in, she ran to her room.

Step 4: What happens after the undesirable interaction occurs? It is critical to understand the entire cycle (before, during, and after) the behavior in question.

THERAPIST: You said she went to her room afterward—why? Do you know what she does there? Are either of them "in trouble"?

PARENT: I think she goes to her room because we used to punish her by sending her there. Whenever she hits him, she loses the iPad for the night. So she didn't get to use it anymore that day. She always says she's going to stop hitting him, but she doesn't seem able to do it.

THERAPIST: What did he do for the rest of the evening?

PARENT: Come to think of it, he used the iPad for the rest of the night. It was longer than the half hour he usually gets, but we feel sorry for him after she hits him.

THERAPIST (as nonjudgmentally as possible): Do you think he has noticed that he gets more iPad time after she hits him?

Step 5: Find out when this behavior does not occur. Sometimes you can learn as much about what happens by figuring out when it doesn't happen. Do they ever play nicely together? This information can be very helpful in choosing the interventions to apply. If a person never behaves poorly in a specific situation, what are the characteristics about that experience that make it different?

THERAPIST: Was there a day this week that they didn't fight about the iPad?

PARENT: Actually, it almost never happens when they visit their grandmother on Tuesdays.

THERAPIST: What is different about their grandmother's house?

PARENT: They have a snack with her and play a board game. They don't get any iPad time.

Step 6: Postgame analysis. When in this cycle could something have happened differently? The purpose of this analysis is to collaborate with the parents to choose interventions.

THERAPIST: Let's look at points along the way when you might have intervened. What do you wish you could do next time?

PARENT: Maybe I could be with my son when he comes home and help him get settled.

THERAPIST: That sounds like a good idea. I also wonder if the kids know whose turn it is and how to transition the iPad. Have you thought about making the rules clearer?

The Three Intervention Moments

In the example we have just gone through, two of the "usual suspects" are at play: digital media and sibling conflict. In this case, you might think about a number of ways to intercede during the three intervention moments: pregame, game, and postgame.

Pregame

Help the parent think about whether there are ways in which the family can be more proactive. Could there be more consistent structure about iPad use? Maybe the children's return from school could be organized in a different way? Or some skills could be taught to both children in terms of delaying gratification and sharing? Maybe the daughter can practice ways, in advance, to manage her brother's predictable grabbing of the iPad that would not get her into trouble. All of these solutions would take less effort and be less time-consuming than dealing with the children when the hitting occurs.

Game

When the hitting starts, the parent can be more intentional in responding. Should going to her room and losing iPad time be the go-to penalty for the daughter? Since the problem recurs almost daily, we can observe that the current strategy is not improving the behavior. Would closer monitoring during the transition time be helpful? Would a discussion with both kids be helpful as the situation is developing? Should the brother's grabbing behavior be examined as a problem in the same way that her hitting him is seen as a difficulty?

Postgame

Planning a more prosocial response, other than hitting, would be useful for the daughter. A number of interventions—environmental (one of them goes to an after-school program, for example), skills-based (learning to share), and reward-based—can be applied. The brother's benefit of extra iPad time should likely be eliminated, despite his victim status. Also, use your knowledge of what is different at the grandmother's house when making suggestions.

This example highlights a way of talking about daily problems that helps identify recurrent difficulties. Worksheet 7.1, "The Usual Suspects," will help you and the caregivers address them.

In the next chapter, we use the steps we have just covered as a framework for addressing four of the main daily struggles: homework, bedtime, eating, and hygiene.

WORKSHEET 7.1

The Usual Suspects

Which of the following are concerns?

- Homework
- Bedtime
- Mealtimes (poor nutrition/hunger)
- Toothbrushing/bathing
- Digital media
- Going to school
- Music, sports, and other extracurricular activities
- Sibling conflict

What might help things go differently?

____

____

____

____

Solutions to try:

1. ____

2. ____

3. ____

4. ____

CHAPTER 8

Daily Struggles

Homework, Bedtime, Eating, and Hygiene

PACT: "C" for "Choose"

Family life with children is rife with opportunities for struggle. Many daily activities lead to stress and conflict. Given that homework, sleeping, eating, and hygiene are regular occurrences, having strategies to manage the typical difficulties that arise for families around these activities is helpful.

Homework

It is rare to find a child or a caregiver who has never been stressed about homework. Though one might question the value of homework (Kohn, 2006), it is a part of childhood and a frequent source of both distress and conflict in families. Many parents describe homework as a catalyst for difficult child behavior and mood issues.

When homework is the culprit, you should ask about the child's routine around it and the attitudes held by family members about its importance. A typical battle, for example, ensues when the child does the "least possible," and the parent believes they are not doing their best. Having a shared agreement about homework, including a time and space in which to accomplish it and a general plan about how it should be done, reduces conflict. Lessening parental anxiety about homework and creating an optimal and intentional plan for the child can prevent a host of difficulties.

When thinking about homework troubles, a central question is: "Is it can't or won't?" (Greene, 1998). Can the child manage after-school work? Maybe the homework level is not right for the child. Maybe the child's attention is spent for the day. Ask the parents: "Is [this] homework a reasonable expectation for your child?" If the child's mental health is at stake, homework may not be the top priority. That said, leaving homework incomplete may also hurt the child's self-esteem, worsen their disconnection from school, or create a backlog of work for the child to contend with. If the parent is uncertain about the child's ability to complete homework, it may be helpful to refer the child for an educational assessment. After many years of unsuccessful homework completion, families sometimes discover that their child has a learning disability that either prevents them from doing the work or makes the work more difficult.

Questions to ask when homework is a source of concern could be:

- How does homework go?
- What is the child's attitude toward homework?
- What is the caregiver's attitude toward homework?
- How much help does the child require to start or complete homework?
- When does the child do homework?
- Where does the child do homework?
- Is homework at the right level for the child?
- Does homework interfere with the child's other activities, and do other activities interfere with homework completion?
- Has the child had psychological or neuropsychological testing?
- Does the child receive special help at school (a 504 plan or an individualized education program)?

After assessing the reasons for the difficulty with homework, and potentially while awaiting the results of testing and school reports, the parents will benefit from your suggestions. Solutions are more successful when they are developed in partnership with the child, the parents, and the school. Some common issues that can be addressed with families include:

1. *Too much time is spent on homework.* When the amount of time spent on homework is markedly out of line with what is reasonable for the child's age or developmental level, recommend that the school issue a "content reduction," which means that the child completes some homework but not as much as the other students. This adjustment is helpful if the child does not need as much repetition to learn something new or is developing homework success and stamina. Sometimes schools will tell their students to stop doing homework after they have tried for a specified amount of time. The National Education Association (2019) generally supports the idea that children should have no more time than 10 minutes multiplied by the grade they are in per night. This means that a seventh grader would have no more than 70 minutes of homework a night.

2. *The full assignment consists of too much work at once.* Though it may not always be obvious, it is overwhelming for some children to complete a whole assignment at once. Divide the homework assignment into more manageable chunks. For example, if a child finds the third-grade writing assignment difficult, they can generate ideas and dictate as the parent scribes (writes). The child can copy the written words later, completing the whole assignment in two steps, rather than having to generate ideas and manage the motor skills required for writing at the same time.

3. *The child lacks stamina or focus.* When the child lacks the ability to complete their homework in one sitting, suggest experimenting with breaks, snacks, and movement. Parents can set a timer (e.g., 10–15 minutes) for work and breaks (5 minutes). However, some children have more difficulty with this approach, because breaks take them out of the mindset of doing work. As with any suggestion, monitor the impact of the change and tailor the intervention to the child.

4. *Scheduling homework is a challenge.* Assess optimal times for the child to complete homework. Some children benefit from having a break after school and starting homework after dinner or after a snack and some downtime. Other kids are more focused on doing homework right after school, so for them continuing directly from the school day is the best option. Or sometimes children participate in many extracurricular activities and begin homework late in the day when they are already fatigued. Review the parameters with the parents so that they can experiment themselves to find the best time.

5. *There is no designated and organized homework space.* Disorganization of the space at home can make working difficult for some children, so having a structured, organized workspace is helpful. A nearby parent, who does not impose their presence on the child, can also keep the child on task and quickly move them through stuck points that arise.

6. *Completing homework at home is challenging.* Doing homework *at* home can be difficult for some children. Help parents figure out the best place to do homework. Often children work better in a structured environment, which may be why homework clubs are such a good option for many families. Other children may prefer a library, a café, their own room, or the kitchen table. Discuss where homework took place when it was achieved most successfully.

7. *The child has weak executive-functioning skills.* Some children lack the organizational skills they need to know what they have to do and how to get started. Parents or teachers can organize homework tasks into a list, which both creates a visual reminder and helps the child recognize what has been completed. Checking off completed tasks on a list can generate a sense of accomplishment and build organizational skills.

8. *The child lacks intrinsic motivation to complete homework.* Caregivers can have a conversation with their child about why they should complete homework, including asking what they hope to get out of it. Caregivers can refer back to previous accomplishments or the feeling of pride their children got from completing an assignment. When a child does not appear to have internal motivation to complete homework, parents can link it to other activities. For example, being told, "You can play Minecraft as soon as you complete your homework." may increase the child's interest in finishing the task. For some older children, parents can talk with them about external reasons for doing homework such as "This is one way that you can show your teachers what you can do."

9. *When rewards would be additionally useful.* If intrinsic motivation is lacking, rewards can be a useful tool. A reminder about something they do want, such as a small prize, might help children get started on their homework. It also pairs homework,

which may be less preferred, with something (the prize) that the child enjoys, which can change the child's feelings about homework.

10. *Homework is too challenging for the child.* Consider recommending a formal evaluation for the child.

11. *Parental pressure increases homework stress and conflict.* Parents contribute to stress about homework when they become more focused on homework completion than the assignment merits, which can happen with optional assignments and extra-credit work or when teachers allow a child to only do what can be completed in a given timeframe. Increase parental self-awareness about any unease that is out of proportion and help them reframe their concern.

Identifying the best ways for children to complete homework, with parent support, leads to feelings of success for both caregivers and children and reduces the conflict accompanying this daily task.

Sleep

Sleep deprivation in children leads to problems in executive functioning, learning, mood management, and behavioral control (Killgore, 2010; Taveras et al., 2017). In addition, the child's sleep can impact the caregivers' sleep, their relationship with their partner, their mood, and the energy needed to manage parenting. Increasing sleep for all family members grants a myriad of preventive benefits across many realms (Mindell & Williamson, 2018). The American Academy of Pediatrics guidelines (Paruthi et al., 2016) suggest these daily parameters for sleep: 10–13 hours, including naps, for preschoolers (3–5 years old); 9–12 hours for school-age children (6–12 years old); and 8–10 hours for teenagers.

The following questions can help assess a child's sleep pattern and routine.

- How does sleep go for this child?
- What are sleep patterns like for this family?
- When is bedtime, ideally, if there is a stated bedtime?
- What is the sleep pattern, including nighttime waking and morning waking?
- How many hours does the child sleep?
- What is the bedtime routine?
- When does the child actually get into bed?
- After the child gets into bed, how long does it take for the child to fall asleep (ease of sleep onset)?
- Does the family co-sleep?
- Are there efforts to postpone bedtime?
- Does the child eat at night?
- Does the child consume caffeine at night?
- Does the child have nighttime enuresis or encopresis?

- Does the child have nightmares or typically report anxiety at night?
- Does the child "sleep" with a phone and have round-the-clock access?
- Does the child fall asleep watching shows, using social media, or texting?
- Does the child rely on a phone as an alarm clock?
- Does the child snore?
- Does the child appear tired even after many hours of sleep?
- Does the child have other sleep anomalies or respiratory issues?
- Has a sleep study been recommended?
- What interventions have been tried (such as relaxation apps or melatonin)?

With this information in mind, formulate your understanding of the problem, and think about the following issues that could be interfering with the child's sleep, including:

1. *The child lacks a regular sleep routine.* Help caregivers build a consistent and healthy sleep routine. It could include a snack, toothbrushing, reading, songs, hugs, and some scripting ("Sleep tight."). Some kids do well with a drink, such as water or herbal tea, as long as it does not lead to the need for bathroom use during the night. Sticking to the nightly routine may be especially important if there has been parent–child conflict, as it serves to reassure the child that the relationship is secure.

2. *The child has an irregular sleep schedule.* Have caregivers establish regular sleep-and-wake times and a quiet room and bed for the child to sleep in.

3. *The child has sleep phase issues.* Similarly, work with the parents to institute regular sleep and wake times. Talk about how late the child sleeps in on nonschool days. The child should not sleep more than an hour later. If the sleep phase is very far off what is healthy, develop a schedule for getting it back on track, which might include waking 30 to 60 minutes earlier each day and then going to bed correspondingly earlier. In severe cases, it is sometimes recommended to shift throughout the day, going to sleep later and later until the sleep phase is where it should be. In these cases, it might be helpful to consult a sleep expert.

4. *The child does not think of their bed as a place just for sleep.* Particularly for children who have trouble falling asleep, encourage the family to create another space in the child's room for reading before bed, if that is something they do. The child can get used to the bed being just for sleeping, rather than for other activities, such as reading or playing games.

5. *The child has trouble relaxing and settling down.* If the child has trouble settling down to a relaxed, sleepy state despite a predictable and calming nighttime routine, teach the parent to use guided meditation and progressive muscle relaxation with their child.

6. *The child's room is not conducive to sleep.* It is surprising how many times you may find that there is not a regular, dark, quiet sleeping space for the child. Blackout curtains

are useful for children whose sleep is very sensitive to light. White noise machines or apps can help if there is distracting ambient noise.

7. *The child may benefit from medical interventions.* If sleep onset or maintenance (waking up in the night) is still difficult even after you have tried these techniques, referring the child to their pediatrician for a sleep study or other medical intervention may be worth trying. If the child has had ongoing respiratory symptoms or is chronically snoring, a referral is especially important since these conditions may indicate medical reasons for the child's sleep challenges.

8. *The child routinely has bad dreams.* When bad dreams or worry about bad dreams are the issue, inquire whether these dreams are linked to real-life concerns or are a signal of increased stress for the child. Sometimes dreams give information about the actual problems going on in the child's life. If the dreams provide insight into why the child is worried, you can address that worry more directly. For example, if a child repeatedly dreams about being seen as "dumb" in school, you can find out if they are struggling academically. Some dreams, such as those about monsters, falling, and being caught in embarrassing situations, are normative experiences for most children, though they may still wish for parental support when they experience them.

9. *Symbolic solutions for bad dreams and worries.* Children can benefit from symbolic solutions for both anxiety overall and bad dreams in particular. These work well for children since they are usually comfortable using their imagination. When the symbolic solution turns into an elongated ritual that must be repeated, then it is not serving its reassuring function and should be discontinued or reconfigured. Examples of symbolic solutions include:

- *Dreamcatchers.* Dreamcatchers are decorated hoops that are thought to inspire good dreams and trap bad ones. Children can make them, or they can be purchased.
- *Worry boxes.* The child symbolically puts concerns from the day away in a decorated real or imagined box. This solution is more powerful if the box is made with the parent. Alternatively, use a well-developed image of a box, in which worries can be placed, with the lid on tightly, locking the box and putting it in a safe place. The caregiver can help the child review what worries to put in the box as part of the bedtime routine.
- *"Monster spray."* The child and caregiver decorate a spray bottle and fill it with water or another solution. As part of the nighttime routine, the parent and child spray and say something like "Monster, monster, stay away."

10. *Nighttime anxiety keeps the child awake.* Many situations cause temporary anxiety that impact sleep. Some examples include school issues, parental conflict, events in the news, friendship issues, and scary reading or visual material consumed before bedtime. When situational anxiety impacts bedtime, find out what the child is fearful of or ruminating about. If the child is focused on a situational concern, work with the family on how to coach the child in the moment to fall asleep, while simultaneously

working with them to address the specific anxiety more directly. If the child is fearful owing to their consumption of scary reading material or internet content right before bedtime, help the child and family identify appropriate before bed materials for reading or watching.

Frequently children have more ongoing anxiety that makes going to sleep alone challenging. When the child has trouble falling asleep on their own because of more general anxiety, create an anxiety hierarchy with planned and gradual exposures to feared situations. The exposure plan should start with an achievable goal for the child and slowly work toward the desired end goal of the child facing their anxiety and going to sleep independently. Before starting any exposure plan, it is important to ascertain what the child is frightened about. A plan for a child who is afraid of the dark would be very different from the plan for a child who has separation anxiety. Figures 8.1 and 8.2 depict models for an exposure plan for two different parents to use with their children. These examples need to be tailored to the needs and skills of the families with whom you are working, taking into account the child's beginning skill level and fears and parent preferences.

Eating

We have all heard about the impact of being "hangry," which suggests a powerful connection between mood, behavior, and hunger. Hunger itself can lead to impaired cognition, poor decision making, and an increase in aggression (Xie et al., 2020). Not only does hunger affect mental health and behavior, so does having poor nutrition (Owen & Corfe, 2017).

Example for the Child Who Has Trouble Sleeping Because They Are in Their Room with the Lights Off

- Child goes into the room briefly during the day with the lights off.
- Child plays in the room during the day with the lights off.
- Child plays sitting near their bed during the day with the lights off.
- Child lies in bed looking at a book during the day with the lights off.
- Child lies in bed looking at a book in bed at night before bedtime.
- Child lies in bed with the lights turned down progressively lower (with a dimmer if available) before bedtime.
- Child lies in bed with the lights turned to the desired darkness level at bedtime for 5 minutes (progressing by 5-minute intervals to 30 minutes).
- Child falls asleep in bed with a night-light or stars on the ceiling (end goal); often total darkness is not the necessary end goal.

FIGURE 8.1. Fear of the dark: Model exposure plan.

Example for a Child Who Has Trouble Falling Asleep without Their Parent Present, and the Parent and/or Child Wants the Child to Sleep with Increased Independence

- Child starts the night in their own bed with the parent sitting at the side of their bed.
- Child closes their eyes and falls asleep with the parent sitting at the side of their bed.
- Child closes their eyes and falls asleep with the parent sitting on a chair near their bed.
- Child closes their eyes and falls asleep with the parent sitting in a chair that is moved (noted by colored tape on the floor) closer to the door each night.
- Child closes their eyes and falls asleep with the parent sitting on a chair that is outside the child's door with the door open.
- Parent comes in and out of the child's room as the child is falling asleep and, over time, gradually increases the intervals between check-ins.
- Parent says good night and the child sleeps on their own (end goal).

FIGURE 8.2. Separation anxiety at night: Model exposure plan.

Positive rituals around food, including regular, healthy mealtimes play a preventive role for children. Just as a bedtime routine is useful for providing structure and well-being for children, so are the family rituals around meals and eating. The title of Miriam Weinstein's 2006 book sums it up: *The Surprising Power of Family Meals: How Eating Together Makes Us Smarter, Stronger, Healthier, and Happier.*

However, there are many obstacles to creating a positive family ritual around meals. Some families eat in front of a screen. Sometimes children come home from school hungry because lunchtime at school can be startlingly short, early in the day, stressful, and oriented around socializing rather than around food. Kids might report that they have not eaten at school owing to a combination of social anxiety and time constraints. When mealtimes or poor eating habits are brought up as difficulties, carefully explore the family's eating patterns. Inquire about patterns of meals and snacks, including both the timing and tenor:

- What is the caregiver's aspirational idea of the family meal versus the real pattern?
- What are mealtimes like?
- Are there patterns or rituals around eating?
- Where and when does the family eat? If they eat at a table, does everyone wait for all family members to sit before they begin?
- Are meals rushed?
- Who prepares the meals?
- What does the family eat? Are there food restrictions due to beliefs or allergies?
- Is the child a picky eater? What do they eat and how do they express their food preferences?
- Are there arguments about eating and trying new foods?
- How stressed is the parent about their child's nutrition?

- Does that stress add to general dysfunction around food?
- Is the pediatrician concerned? Is the child growing appropriately?
- Do other activities accompany mealtimes (such as doing homework, watching TV, using phones)?
- Are meals a trigger for conflict?
- Do the siblings compete for attention during meals?
- Are there different meals for each family member?
- Are table manners important to the caregivers?
- Do the children have a reasonable transition to the new activity of the meal?
- Is there conversation during meals?

With the answers to this list of questions in mind, there are a number of ways to intervene around child eating and family mealtime problems. Some of the following examples illustrate the common difficulties families experience during mealtimes and potential solutions:

1. *Assess what makes the mealtime challenging.* Address concerns in a targeted way. Not eating together may be part of another problem, such as significant parent–child conflict or overscheduling, which are addressed elsewhere in this book. However, if this is a more limited concern, then there may be straightforward solutions, such as building a ritual, setting a scheduled mealtime, reducing noise, or managing sitting expectations.

2. *Mealtime routines are lacking.* Mealtime routines can be improved in a number of ways.

   a. *Mealtime predictability or consistency is insufficient:* Establishing routines can help improve mealtimes. Having regular meals at predictable times is a good start. Since many children are in extracurricular activities until late in the evening, foregoing dinner, have a predictable where, when, and what will happen for each meal and snack, even when family members may need to eat "on the run." Caregivers should give children food before they are so hungry that their hunger affects their mood, so planning ahead is required.

   b. *There are few rituals that make mealtimes special or differentiated.* If you discover that there is no regular meal pattern, recommend to parents that they create meal rituals. Saying grace for families who believe in the practice can be a healthy way to start a meal. If not, there are other consistent ways to start a meal. Everyone can bring food items to the table, or families can have scripted conversations such as gratitude practice, telling jokes, or answering questions from "conversation starter" card sets. Knowing what to expect and having predictability in the eating experience help children look forward to meals. Special treats, such as "Taco Tuesdays" or "Ice Cream Fridays," reduce guesswork and begging for particular meal items.

   c. *There is no clear start and end time.* As part of the meal pattern, systematize how meals start and end. Make it explicit when the child can leave the table and what they are expected to do next, which can be taking dishes to the sink, doing homework, taking a bath, or enjoying a fun activity (such as watching a show). The parents may also need to alert the child about when meals start. For example, if the child is working on homework, the parent can give them a time warning: "In about 5 minutes I need you to set the table for dinner." This warning suggests that the parent does not expect the child to stop what they are doing immediately, and also involves the child in a meal preparation activity for a potentially smoother transition.

3. *The child has trouble sitting through a meal.* For children who have trouble sitting through an entire meal, work on images to help them feel more grounded in the chair, such as "glue that holds them in their chair" or having a foundation "like a tree with deep roots." Help parents to develop realistic expectations for how long a child should sit that considers both their developmental level and the individual characteristics of the child. Find out whether the child has little trouble sitting in restaurants and at other people's houses. If caregivers recognize that the difficulty happens primarily at home, perhaps they can worry less about it.

4. *Mealtime feels rushed or chaotic.* Establish a relaxing meal environment, which may mean reducing rushing through meals and pairing meals with other pleasant stimuli. Relaxing music in the background can be considered, especially if noise and chaos during meals have been part of the problem.

5. *The child does not engage in conversation.* Sometimes the conversations during the mealtime work against successful dining experiences, whether they are intensive conversations above the child's head and exceed their attention span or are inquisitions about the child's life at school. Instead, have parents bring up more neutral topics that are of interest to the children. Suggest that caregivers make statements that they think children might respond to, rather than demanding a response with a question. Examples might include, "Hey, I saw an ad for the new Marvel movie today. I think it comes out in about a month"; or "The dog did the funniest thing today. She went out and buried herself in the snow. I got some good pictures."

6. *The child is a picky eater.* Children have almost double the number of taste buds as adults do (McElwain, 2019), which may be why they have more food aversions. Help the parents understand the reason behind their child's pickiness. If a child is reluctant to try new foods, help the parents to introduce them more than once. Children may need multiple exposures to new foods before they feel confident enough to eat them. Help parents create a narrative about a food they were reluctant to try as children but wound up enjoying as adults. Recommend that parents introduce new foods one at a time so that the child is not overwhelmed and have them take one lick or bite of the food each time. If a child needs a more involved program, try this formula for trying new foods (with several trials at each step): Look, touch, smell, kiss, lick, bite, and finally eat.

7. *Caregivers' affect regarding the child's picky eating increases mealtime stress.* Parents can become frustrated about their child's picky eating. Some families resort to and

resent making two or more different meals each night. Offering "deconstructed" meals allows the pickier eater to have the components they enjoy without the family having to cook another meal. An example might be tacos with toppings that are not assembled, so that each person can choose the ingredients they want.

8. *The child expresses dislike for the food in a disrespectful way.* Children sometimes complain about the foods presented to them, worsening the mealtime atmosphere. Typical child comments about meals may include "That's gross," "Ew," or "I'm not eating that." Identify appropriate responses to these comments, such as "You don't have to eat it all, but I'd like you to . . ." or "When you don't want to eat something, you can say, 'No, thank you.' " Recommend that parents involve children in making the meal since children are often more invested in eating a meal when they have a role in creating it. They can help grow food, choose meals, grocery shop, and prepare food.

9. *The child eats snacks without permission.* Sometimes conflict arises because children choose or sneak snacks that have not been approved by the parents. The first steps may be to figure out what foods the parents consider nutritious (that the child also will eat) and then make them easily accessible and convenient. Determine whether the child is actually hungry and needs more snacks. Put nutritious, perishable and nonperishable food options within the child's reach. Similarly, recommend that the parents be more intentional with their choices of food purchases. Why have candy in the cupboard if it is not permitted? Reducing the purchase of foods that parents deem undesirable can help to reduce conflict. The environment can be organized to increase or decrease the snacking of particular foods; for example, putting approved food on the table will increase the likelihood that it is chosen as a snack.

Sometimes parents label sneaking snacks in ways that increase negative affect; for example, some caregivers call this behavior "stealing." In those situations, work with the parents to reframe their thinking about it, while recognizing that they can work to improve the child's behavior. Sneaking food and hoarding food can also be related to other diagnoses, such as reactive attachment disorder or eating disorders. In those instances, a clinician skilled in working with those diagnoses will have appropriate recommendations.

10. *The parents are concerned about the child's weight.* If the child's weight (either overweight or underweight) is a concern, encourage the parents to follow up with their pediatrician. With specific recommendations from the child's doctor, you can tailor your program according to their advice. If the parents are very worried and the pediatrician is not concerned, work with them to manage their anxiety and expectations. Receiving medical reassurance can reduce caregivers' anxieties.

11. *Messaging about weight and bodies in the family causes issues.* Help parents consider how they talk about food and body size with or around their children. Discussions about food can focus on having a strong, healthy body rather than about having a different body size.

12. *Using food as a reward or consequence.* Be thoughtful about using food as a reward or consequence. Some families can use food appropriately in this way without it causing additional distress or discord. But if food is a hot-button issue for parents or family members, find other reinforcers.

13. *Family rules about food are nonexistent or unworkable.* Help caregivers keep food rules workable and reasonable. For example, is dessert earned by eating other foods? One family uses the concept of "dessert eligible," which is based on balancing food choices and removes some arguments about desserts and healthy foods.

Hygiene

There is actually a word for the fear of bath time—*ablutophobia*—and many children seem to have it. Bath time, washing hands and faces, hair brushing, and toothbrushing provoke regular family battles. These daily hygiene requirements are hard to accomplish without the cooperation of all involved. Toothbrushing, in particular, is important for children's health, and it is very difficult to brush the teeth of an uncooperative person or to teach a child how to do this well on their own (Marshman et al., 2016). Disagreements about how often kids should bathe and brush their teeth are commonplace.

When these daily hygiene situations cause difficulties for the family, ask the caregiver these questions:

- Is there a routine for hand washing?
- Is there a routine for hair brushing?
- Is there a routine for bathing?
- Is there a routine for toothbrushing?
- What is the timing for these activities?
- What are the child's and caregivers' views about hygiene?
- How much help does the child need to accomplish these activities?
- What happens when the child does not complete the activity?
- Has the child received feedback from peers or adults about their hygiene?
- Is there sensory sensitivity (difficulty with tags in clothing or heightened responses to different textures, tastes, or sounds)?

The following list includes some common difficulties concerning hygiene and suggestions to assist with hygiene routines:

1. *There is no predictable hygiene routine:* Help parents create and utilize regular and predictable schedules for these activities. They will go more smoothly if they are done daily at the same time.

2. *The child dislikes the options given.* Have parents give the child choices when possible; families can then negotiate which ones are realistic. The timing of bathing, or the choice of showering versus bathing, or the bath products that they use can all be reasonable options to discuss. If the child uses more shampoo or another product than the parent would like, can they come to a reasonable solution, such as purchasing less-expensive products?

3. *There is bath time anxiety.* Find out if the child has any worries about taking a bath. If so, address them directly. Have the parents let the child know when bath time will begin and end.

4. *Parents do not model hygiene behavior for their children.* Children benefit from modeling of good hygiene behavior. Recommend that caregivers model the hygiene behavior that they desire for their children. There are also readily available YouTube videos of same age peers engaging in most of the daily hygiene activities.

5. *Stalling.* When stalling occurs because the hygiene routine leads to bedtime, recommend that bathing and toothbrushing be followed with preferred activities by scheduling them earlier in their nighttime routine.

6. *Sensory sensitivities.* Sensory factors can make hygiene activities difficult. Educate parents about the sensory aspects of these activities and find ways to make them more comfortable or enjoyable. Different flavors of toothpaste may be available, including chocolate and strawberry, for children who dislike the regular flavors of toothpaste. Some families use ice pops in the shower as distracting sensory input. Children can also play with shaving cream in the bathroom. The sensory input can be enjoyable, which can help shower-reluctant children tolerate and even enjoy showers. If sensory issues are a long-standing concern, consider an occupational therapy evaluation.

7. *Hygiene activities are no fun.* Make hygiene more fun! Bathing toys, colored water, or a bubble bath for younger children can reduce bathing reluctance. Teach parents to help younger children role play these hygiene scenarios with a doll or stuffed animal. For older children, listening to music or a particular song can be paired with a shower as a way to suggest an appropriate length of shower time and to increase enjoyment.

8. *Communication about hygiene activities is fraught.* Role play with parents how to talk with their child about hygiene and hygiene activities realistically but without inducing overwhelming shame. Discourage caregivers from questioning children about their hygiene when they are certain that they have neglected it. Sometimes parents ask children about toothbrushing in a way that will perpetuate an unfortunate dynamic: They ask if the child brushed their teeth, they then check if the toothbrush is wet, and finally feel angry that the child lied. When this dynamic is in play, suggest that the caregiver watch the child engage in the activity.

These approaches are useful in dealing with the four daily struggles outlined in this chapter. In the next chapter we discuss other common problems that lead to arguments at home: digital media; going to school; music, sports, and other extracurricular activities; and sibling conflict.

CHAPTER 9

Other Common Problems That Lead to Frequent Arguments

Digital Media, Going to School, Extracurricular Activities, and Sibling Conflict

Strategies for Addressing These Predictable Subjects of Arguments

These "usual suspects" occur regularly in family life and frequently cause enough challenges that they are brought into the therapist's office. We have detailed interventions for all of them, as they are likely to present as issues in parent guidance.

Digital Media

Digital media provides a significant source of conflict between parents and children. Since the COVID-19 pandemic, more time on electronic devices has become the norm and has become required for many school and work tasks. Caregivers often ask their parent guidance therapist about how to get their child to make nonelectronic choices for their spare time and about the number of hours the child should be using these tools. We have yet to hear a parent say, "My children aren't on their screens enough." Limiting screen time and the use of social media can be necessary for some children, given research on the impact of screen time (Domingues-Montanari, 2017) and the effects of social media (Karim et al., 2020) on children. The American Academy of Child and Adolescent Psychiatry (2020) links screen time to physical health issues, sleep problems, and mental health concerns and recommends that most children decrease their daily usage.

In the early days of our careers, before the advent of smartphones and tablets, parents used to ask us if they should put a television in their child's room. Our answer was typically no, because having their own TV would interfere with the child's sleep and be more isolating than watching a show in a common family area. Now nearly every child, by virtue of having a phone, tablet, or laptop, can immediately have a TV in their room. The following questions can help you think carefully about this issue:

- How does the child use their screen time? What is the child doing on their phone or other devices?
- How much do the caregivers know about what their child is doing on their devices?
- Does the child have a tablet or a cell phone of their own?
- What are the family rules and attitudes about digital media?
- Is there a structure to the day involving screen use?
- Do the caregivers and children agree about the family's use of digital media?
- Have family members thrown or deliberately destroyed devices?
- Is screen time used as a reward?
- Is removal of screen time used frequently to encourage better behavior? Is there follow-through?
- Given the use of screens for school, for family and friend content, and for free time, is it realistic to remove devices for this child?
- Do the caregivers use their child's phone to stay in touch with or track their child, making it difficult to take the phone away?
- What could the child be doing in place of screen time?
- Does the child become distressed by content on their phone or other device?
- Do the caregivers struggle with keeping their own device use manageable?
- Do caregivers and their children ever engage together on devices?
- What nonelectronic activities bring the family together?

After assessing the issues around electronics use, there are a number of ways to intervene. Here are some common issues and possible solutions:

1. *Parents have no clear expectations.* Develop clear family expectations around screen use. Therapists can help parents understand how intentional planning can prevent mental health issues and remediate problems that exist around electronics usage. This can include charging the phones and tablets in the caregivers' room or in a neutral location or having children surrender their devices to parents at a specific time each night. Another useful expectation involves requiring that caregivers have the passwords to access the child's accounts.

The American Academy of Pediatrics (2021) offers a guide to creating a family media plan, which helps the family come to shared agreements about what kinds of shows to watch, when, and how much to watch. When use of electronics is a component of the family stress, we recommend that you help the family create such a plan.

2. *There is not enough device-free time.* Help families create device-free time for parents and children. In general, have caregivers model the use of devices they wish their children would adopt. Many parents, for example, are unable to charge their phones in another room or take a break from their own screens to interact with their children. You

may get clues about the parents' usage based on how they behave with their phones during your sessions.

Encourage families to have fun together, with and without their devices. Identify shows and games for the family to enjoy together. Develop a list of ways for families and children to spend time that do not involve screens. This list can be posted somewhere prominent, such as the refrigerator, and kids can refer back to it.

3. *Device removal is overused as a penalty.* For some families, minimizing the conflict around how much screen time children are allowed may include reducing the use of phone removal as the go-to punishment. Come up with other possibilities for consequences, if they choose to use them, that make sense and are workable.

4. *The child is young and wants or has a personal device.* How old is old enough for a personally owned tablet or smartphone? Consider, with the parents, when it is appropriate to purchase these devices for their children. Help them think through what they will be used for. Tablets can belong to the whole family rather than being the sole property of an individual child. Having a landline will allow the child to reach and be reached by friends without having their own phone.

5. *Parents do not know what children are doing on their devices.* Encourage caregivers to be familiar with the content of the shows and games children engage with on their own. Refer parents to guides such as Common Sense Media and GamerDad that can help families discern the content and appropriateness of what kids are doing on their devices. A new onset of some symptoms can sometimes be related to device content. One patient with anxiety was watching horror movies, which was markedly improved when their parent discovered and limited what they were watching. Children may sometimes express that they enjoy scary content, even when they are distressed by it, making the decision of when to limit it challenging for parents. We recommend erring on the side of limiting content, especially when it is not age appropriate, for anxious or depressed children. Have families make a space for computer use in a public area of the house to encourage monitoring of online activities.

6. *Media safety is poor.* Help caregivers teach media safety. One positive reference for girls is *A Smart Girl's Guide: Digital World: How to Connect, Share, Play, and Keep Yourself Safe* (Anton, 2017).

CASE STUDY: How Much Are Too Much Digital Media?

In working with a set of divorced parents, EB was reminded of the importance of understanding the specifics of the family "rules" and looking at the whole picture before suggesting strategies. The divorced parents of a 10-year-old boy sought parent guidance to manage their son's temper tantrums. During the assessment, the father reported that there were no meltdowns at his home. He believed that meltdowns at the mother's home were due to her strict rules limiting video games, which served as a coping strategy for the boy. The mother nodded, seeming to agree. When asked more specifically about meltdowns at her house, she reported that whenever her son was asked to stop playing video games, he became upset. At this point in the assessment, EB had her own guesses about how much game time there was in each house. She guessed that the mother allowed about 15-to-30 minutes a day of video game time. Instead, the mother reported 5–6 hours of screen time daily. When the father was asked, he said that he allowed 15 hours a day of video game time on a weekend. There were no behavioral outbursts at the father's house because no limits were set. The boy was required to engage in more activities at his mother's house, such as eating dinner without playing video games, leaving the house for walks, showering, and getting dressed.

In this case, getting a clear view of both parents' perspectives was important. Figuring out how to intervene required an understanding of the rules at both homes, a shared understanding of expectations, and getting both parents on board to help build coping skills. Though there is no "right" answer about the exact amount of time a preteen should spend on games, parent guidance depends on bringing all of these data to the table.

Going to School

Parents often ask, "Why does my (young) child get up at 6:00 A.M. every Saturday but have trouble waking at 7:30 A.M. on school days?" With a little perspective taking, we can recognize that we all wake up more readily for desired events. In the context of trying to develop a new morning routine, with an incentive to get up and be ready to be on time for school, one elementary school student said, "I don't want to be at school on time. It starts when I get there. I don't miss anything. When I get there early, it's boring. We are just waiting for others to arrive."

When a child who previously went to school easily starts dragging their feet about going to school, dig deeper. When working with this usual suspect in particular, advise parents to try to figure out the *why* before guiding them on *how* to manage this new avoidance. You may find that there is something stressful going on at school, such as bullying, a conflict with teachers, an academic struggle, or a friendship dilemma. When talking about getting to school, find out how the family's process for getting ready goes both aspirationally and actually. Solutions are more effective when they target the specific issue.

Tardiness and school attendance can be challenging and intractable issues. The following list includes some examples and suggestions to address them.

1. *Assess the reasons for difficulties in going to school.* Address the individual issue(s) in a targeted way. You can help the parent devise an intervention plan around the reasons for the avoidance. If it is school stress, sometimes encouraging the parent to talk to the teacher, who can serve as an ally, about the child's feelings can be remarkably helpful. If

there is a bullying situation or an academic weakness, address these problems directly. If the child's concerns are exaggerated, help the parent to alter the way the child thinks about and experiences the school environment with the following ideas:

- The child may not feel connected with the teacher or feel that the teacher likes them. Coach parents to speak with their child about their feelings regarding their teacher. During this conversation, parents should not try to argue the child out of their feelings. The purpose of this conversation is to uncover underlying concerns.
- Parents can talk with the teacher about the fact that their child is not feeling comfortable in school, and see if they can enlist the teacher to help. They should not share feelings that the child would not want shared. For example, they should avoid saying, "My child does not like you and thinks that you do not like her. Is there anything we can do about that?" Instead, they might say, "My child is struggling to feel comfortable in school. She does really well when she feels connected to her teacher. Might there be ways you could get her involved, such as letting her be a helper when she first comes in in the morning? That might increase her sense of connection."
- Be aware of state laws regarding bullying. If bullying is a concern, parents will need to strategize with their children. Sometimes children accurately assess that directly addressing bullying will worsen the situation. Schools can also be powerful allies in handling bullying. Help parents advocate with the school staff around solutions, such as creating distance between the children, reducing opportunities for bullying to occur through better monitoring, and potentially engaging in restorative justice activities, if the child is comfortable with these ideas.
- Additional tutelage both in or outside of school can address academic weaknesses. However, academic weaknesses may need to be fully assessed through testing, and parents may need guidance on the best ways to implement the recommendations from testing.

2. *The mornings are difficult.* If the child struggles with getting ready for school, you can help the parent to implement a more effective structure and routine, including:

- Get the child started earlier. For getting to school and other early morning activities, parents worry about the amount of sleep that their child has each night, which often leads them to wake the child up at the latest possible minute. While concerns about sleep are laudable, this pressure creates a very tight timeframe. Reliably adding 15–20 minutes allows a buffer and a more relaxed, flexible, and collaborative morning routine.
- Alternatively, if the caregiver is willing, they can allow the child to get a little more sleep but recognize that they may have to do some morning tasks, such as getting the lunch box and backpack ready, or preparing the child's shoes by untying the double knot left over from the day before.
- Encourage the parent to get up earlier than they usually do. This reduces the time pressure on the parent, whether they use the time for self-care (meditation, reading, exercise, eating) or to begin some tasks, such as getting dressed themselves, making breakfast and lunch, and preparing for the day. If the parent uses the extra

time to get ready themself, they can more effectively monitor the child's progress toward the goal of getting out the door on time.

- In designing the morning routine, help the parent assess the child's ability, both developmentally and emotionally, to complete getting ready tasks independently. Parents may focus on the child's age. "He's 7 years old, shouldn't he be dressing himself?" Helping the parent concentrate less on these generic expectations and more on figuring out what the child has been able to do and can do is important. Though children may be physically able to put their pants on themselves, it may be emotionally harder after just waking up and facing the stress of the daily separation from parents. Gradually encouraging more independence through shaping causes less parental frustration and will lead to a more positive routine.
- In order to make the morning go more quickly, recommend that parents and children complete as much preparation as possible the day before. Without the time pressure, parents can more effectively include the child in making decisions for the day and can improve the child's executive functioning skills. The night before, the parent and child can choose the outfit, check the next day's schedule to find out what is needed (such as sneakers or library books), check the backpack and homework folder, place the backpack and coat near the door, and pack lunch. To speed up the morning routine, some parents allow their children to wear the next day's clothes to bed.
- Find out if the mornings have been regularly stressful. Examples of difficult moments can include parents becoming angry because the child refuses to get out of bed and the parent resorting to pulling the child out of the bed. If these negative patterns exist, it will be especially important to develop a more positive ritual to wake the child up. Sometimes this ritual can include kisses, tickles, jokes, songs, or reading a book. Be mindful of what will work for this particular child and know that it will change as the child gets older. JDS used to wake her younger child up by quietly having him move over in his bed so that she could snuggle with him as he woke up. As he got older, that ritual was definitely out. However, the routine shifted to her coming in to his room, saying "move over," and him jokingly spreading out to make it impossible for her to join him, all without opening his eyes but sometimes with a mischievous smile. All kids benefit from a fun start to the day, but it will be especially important to establish a ritual if the family is used to a negative start.
- Once a routine has been intentionally devised, it helps to have cues to remind the children and parents of the morning plan. Ask the family to create a checklist with visual cues. Time reminders, such as "In 5 minutes it will be time to put shoes on," can also help the child and parent stay on track and help the child transition between the getting ready activities.
- Teach the parents to use bridging activities to help the morning go more smoothly. This option often motivates the child to complete the required tasks more efficiently. Be careful that the chosen activity fits into the time slot. As one parent said, "We don't have time to make a glitter tiara before school!" If the parent allows the child to watch a television show, assess that this choice fits into the time left, as children can become very upset about turning off a 22-minute show at the 16-minute

mark. In addition, some children simply have more, not less, difficulty transitioning from digital media to less-preferred activities, which means that for them the remaining time before school should be spent in a different way.

- One successful intervention for some children is to get to school early, which allows them to play in the playground or have some fun time with friends. Another option that is motivating is teaming up with another parent and child and arriving early for playtime together. Ironically, getting up early to both reduce the time pressure and to have a desirable activity before the school day starts is often a successful intervention to recommend to parents. Though children sometimes claim they do not want to be first student to arrive at school, they can enjoy it once they have experienced it a few times.

3. *The child does not feel connected with people at school.* If the child feels disconnected at school, the school staff can be powerful allies in building connections by greeting the child every morning. It does not have to be an elaborate greeting, but it should be one in which the staff conveys they are excited to see this individual child. The greeter can be a teacher, a guidance counselor, or administrative staff person. There are anecdotes about teachers creating individual handshakes for each child in their class, videos of which can be found online.

4. *More severe school avoidance.* More severe school refusal can occur when children have significant anxiety about attending school. For these situations, graduated exposure programs can work well. Some children do well with going to school for short periods of time, with the time increasingly getting longer. Others benefit from being able to spend time in the guidance office and using that as a starting point. They can then spend some time in class but return to the guidance office without leaving school. Build an individualized hierarchy for returning to a more normative school schedule.

Music, Sports, and Other Extracurricular Activities

Extracurricular activities, though they are meant to be fun and instructive, can lead to family stress and conflict. Parents feel pressured to encourage their children to take up hobbies in order to build skills, develop a talent, reduce sedentary screen time, and increase socialization. However, sometimes the costs outweigh the benefits. An internet search quickly produces multiple queries from desperate parents: "How do I get my child to practice?" "How do you motivate an unmotivated child?" Practice in hobbies, such as sports, music, theater, or academic activities, can inspire similar battles as those that arise homework. Speak with parents about their motivations for encouraging the child to continue in an activity, which may include more built-in time for the parent to spend at work, making connections with other parents and having social time at the sidelines, continuing family traditions, feeling competitive with other families, wishing for the child to excel, and giving the child a competitive advantage on their college applications. Be aware that, in some parts of the country and among some subgroups, there is a lot of spoken or unspoken pressure around these activities.

Helpful questions to ask include:

- How does the activity and practice happen?
- Who chose it?
- How much parent and child investment is there in this activity?
- What is the child's mood during practice?
- What is the impact of the teacher or coach?
- What is the culture and stress level of the activity?
- Is the child placed at the right level?
- What are the other children who participate in the activity like?
- Are there built-in issues of unfairness?

Some issues to consider and suggestions to help parents make proactive decisions about hobbies and related practice could include the following:

1. *Help the parent assess the pros and cons of each activity for the child.* If the child has no hobbies, you may want to help the parent direct the child to try various activities to find an interest. If the chosen hobbies pose a problem, you may ask if there is another activity that would be a better match. Many youth trade a team sport, such as soccer, which requires attending to multiple stimuli at once, for an individual sport, such as running or swimming, if the complexity of the team sport is too challenging.

2. *Is the child overscheduled?* By overscheduled we mean that the number of events or time it takes to complete the activities appears to be causing stress to the child and overshadows opportunities for free time, relaxation, or even the activities of daily life, such as eating, sleeping, playdates, and homework completion. Sometimes teams have practices that go past the child's bedtime. If the parents and child want to continue this activity, help them creatively develop work-arounds, such as eating in the car or getting extra help to complete homework, that can decrease the stress. Consider whether the child's pattern of behavioral or mental health concerns is linked to their hobby.

3. *Is a teacher or coach a bad match for this child?* When the adults involved in a child's activity cause struggles, help the parent assess the optimal match in a coach or teacher for their child. The person with the most exacting style may promote marked improvements for some children, inspiring more practice. If, however, the child feels downtrodden or is berated by a teacher, a warmer, more relational teacher may be a better fit. Some youth may want to engage in the activity simply for fun, which some teachers can support, but others struggle with. Parents often do not consider ways to make a hobby and the teacher associated with it a better match.

4. *The child and parent disagree about practice.* Help parents consider what constitutes good practice. With musical instruments and sports, practice is critical to improvement and is an important aspect of participation. Teaching children to have the discipline to practice is valuable beyond the benefit of the hobby. Parents often resort to threats and bribes to make practice happen, rather than helping the child take ownership over their

own improvement. Seeing the link between improvement and effort can inspire kids in many arenas (Dweck, 2008). When children are told to practice for a certain amount of time and are rewarded for doing so or penalized for failing to do so, practice becomes rote and obligatory rather than a journey toward improvement or enjoyment. Battles regarding practice are a sign of trouble for the hobby.

5. *The child struggles with competition.* Competition can cause stress for some children. Find out how the child manages winning and losing, seating placement in music ensembles, positions on their team, disappointing role assignments in the school musical, and other signs of the child's successful or less successful experiences. In addition to encouraging the child to practice the hobby, the parent can assist the child in developing scripts for themselves in predictable situations that occur (e.g. "I'll get it next time"). Encourage the parent to develop some normative automatic social scripts with the child, such as "Nice match" or "Good shot" in tennis, or "Good game" at the end of board games, regardless of the outcome.

Sibling Conflict

Sibling interactions are a regular source of discussion in parent guidance work. Though siblings can get along well, sibling battles can also be a source of family stress. There is the fight over where they sit on the couch; hitting or kicking or simply touching each other in the car; insulting and demeaning each other; comparing seemingly identical items (e.g., servings of ice cream); and demanding "equal" treatment, such as the same bedtime even though one child is older. Children might define a situation as unfair and become upset by it, even when it is out of the parents' control. For example, one child might get angry that they did not get the goody bag that their sibling got, despite not attending the party where the bags were doled out.

Competitive patterns can be subtly encouraged by parents or teachers who, in an effort to call forth good behavior, say, "So and so is sitting nicely, why can't you?" We have worked with families who have races to see which child gets ready more quickly, increasing rivalry. We have also worked with the child who is more often seen as "the good kid" asking, "Was I good?" in the context of sibling misbehavior. In your interventions with parents, identify patterns of sibling behavior and work to help them encourage more cooperative and less competitive sibling relationships. Harmonious sibling relationships have been correlated with fewer internalizing and externalizing problems as well as an increased sense of competence (Buist & Vermande, 2014). Make certain that your interventions do not put siblings at odds or make it advantageous to be the one who is not doing well. For example, if you use rewards, you can create a system in which siblings help each other or in which both children work toward personal goals.

Here are some questions to ask to assess how to intervene with sibling concerns:

- Do conflicts between siblings become physically dangerous?
- How do the siblings in the family interact?

- What are the family attitudes and expectations around sibling interactions?
- Do they realistically and reasonably resolve conflicts on their own and, if so, how?
- Do they spend any positive time together? If so, what do they do?
- Do siblings respect each other's private time and property?

We provide some examples of problematic sibling dynamics, with some suggestions to help the families you are working with to shift the patterns:

1. *Intervene early.* Fatigued parents often suggest "Work it out yourselves" despite the clear power and size differences between their children. Even when siblings are enjoying time together, sibling play might end on a bad note because parents let them play together until something goes wrong. Parents find it difficult to end a positive sibling interaction since it helps them to complete tasks or enjoy a break. Why would you end something that is going well? Suggest to the parents with whom you are working that even when siblings seem to be playing well, periodic check-ins are helpful. If there are no check-ins and sibling play always ends on a sour note, then it colors the way the siblings perceive each other. If an interaction is going poorly, it is unlikely to simply be resolved on its own.

2. *One child provokes the other.* Help parents notice what we call the "jack-in-the-box" effect, which is when one child is predictably winding up their sibling with repeated jabs until the sibling "pops" with explosive behavior. When poking a sibling's weakness, there is a predictable enjoyment in successfully provoking the anger response, especially if it leads to the sibling getting in trouble for reacting. Help parents recognize and disrupt these patterns, including through discussions with both children. If it continues, help parents monitor more effectively and address the child who is engaging in provocation. Caregivers can reduce the time the children spend together and take the fun out of the "jack-in-the-box."

3. *Car ride conflict.* Car rides can be challenging when siblings are engaged in physical altercations while a parent is driving. Parents can think ahead about making car rides more enjoyable, including making a plan for the ride, such as having snacks for the children or an audiobook. A fair system, planned ahead of time, for where children should sit in the car can also increase the likelihood of a successful ride.

4. *Roughhousing ends in tears or arguments.* There are families whose children regularly engage in fighting games, such as wrestling and nerf gun battles, that predictably end in tears or arguments. If these games result in actual fighting, crying, and family disruption, be selective about the content or length of playtime or place the toys in places that encourage outdoor or more limited play. In general, while these games with siblings often start as consensual fun games, they rarely end well.

5. *Siblings dislike each other:* Sometimes siblings are stuck in negative patterns of thought about each other. Help the parent to assist their children in making a cognitive shift, namely that there is something beneficial, interesting, or likable about their

sibling. Sometimes children can be helped to select gifts or souvenirs for their siblings, which builds perspective taking and good will. Sometimes the dynamic can change when a younger child enters school and other students provide a new perspective on their sibling. When there is a significant age difference, some families have allowed older siblings to practice babysitting, for pay or not, with the younger child.

6. *Sibling competition*. Shifting from competitive sibling dynamics to cooperative ones can be assisted with projects and games. Sherif and colleagues (1961) conducted an experiment with children at summer camp ("Robber's Cave"), which showed that it is easy to form a fierce competition among children when there are limited resources. These authors changed the relationships among the campers by finding problems that they needed to solve together. It is likely that, when engaged in joint projects, siblings will also alter their behavior in positive ways. This could include incentives that need to be earned together, or a task such as choosing or making a gift for the parent. There are a number of cooperative board games currently on the market that families can enjoy, for example, Forbidden Island, Castle Panic, and Pandemic, to name a few. A colleague once employed an intervention with a pair of siblings who struggled to get along. They set up a cooperative project that they worked on at separate times; one would go into the room to work on it at one time and the other would go into the room at a later time, look at what the sibling did, and continue the project. They successfully completed a project together, without interacting during the entire process. This intervention created a positive shift in their relationship.

We hope that this review of the usual suspects in parent–child conflict, and our potential solutions for managing them, will help in clinical practice with families. The next part addresses behavioral interventions, an essential item in the clinician's parent guidance toolbox.

PART IV

Making the Most of Your Behavioral Interventions

Behavioral interventions, including creating formal reward systems, educating caregivers about reinforcement and punishment, and looking for patterns in behavior that can be adjusted are frequently used tools for the parent guidance expert. You need to be well versed in these techniques, as you will be called upon to create behavioral plans, determine why they may not be working, and tweak them. The chapters in this section help you set a family up for success in effectively utilizing behavioral interventions.

Veruca Salt's entitled refrain in Roald Dahl's *Charlie and the Chocolate Factory*, "I want it now . . ." rings true for many parents. Veruca Salt may epitomize the strength of a reward system. She demanded and her father provided what she wanted, reinforcing her difficult behavior. Her simpering father was not prepared for the extinction burst when he tried to limit the reinforcement, and he quickly gave in to her. He needed the support of a parent guidance expert who could coach him through the challenges of undoing the inadvertent reinforcement of his daughter's demands.

The chapters in this section focus on factors that create an optimal situation for using rewards and consequences, and then discusses using them. You will teach families to communicate directives effectively and to implement behavioral strategies, and in the process, you will also strengthen the caregivers' awareness of the ways in which they respond ineffectively.

CHAPTER 10

Commands, Praise, and Feedback

This chapter identifies ways to improve the likelihood that children will meet parental expectations and follow directives. Children respond to communications in individualized ways that are heavily influenced by the ongoing patterns and relationships between them and their caregivers. An important aspect of parent guidance is teaching caregivers how their communication impacts ongoing patterns.

Communicating Instructions Effectively

Is the Child's Attention on the Command?

In reviewing communications with parents, assess whether messages are delivered when the children are paying attention. Communications cannot be effective if they are not seen or heard by the intended receiver. Often caregivers are frustrated when their children do not follow their commands, even when the directives are given from different rooms or floors or while the parent is facing the sink doing dishes. Parents improve the effectiveness of their communications by not talking to their child from far away (as in the parent who is downstairs yelling for a child who is upstairs to get dressed) but instead talking to them when they are nearby. Teach caregivers to engage in conversations in the same room as their child, to make eye contact, without being distracted by an electronic device, and to make sure they have the attention of the person to whom they are speaking. If the parent is uncertain about whether their message was received, they can ask the child to repeat it back.

Eliminating Ineffective Commands

Interventions are generally more effective the closer you remain to the person with whom you are intervening. Many parents make a demand, such as "put your toys away," and then leave the room to engage in their own tasks before the chore has been completed. When the parent leaves, the child may return to what they had been doing, essentially becoming distracted from complying with or ignoring the parent's request. Problematic patterns arise when children become used to ignoring parents' commands.

It may be helpful to ask parents about how they communicate instructions to their children, and when attempts to communicate do and do not work well. If children ignore the parent's directions, explore further. Is the request reasonable? Are there too many commands at once? Does the child understand them? Are commands typically delivered multiple times before the child is expected to follow the command (Barkley, 2013)? If parents find themselves asking too many times for something to be done, then the pattern for the child may become completing the task only after being asked 14 times, or only when the parent is frustrated and starts screaming. Instructions should be delivered with a serious tone of voice and facial expression if they are to be understood (Barkley, 2013).

In addition, work with parents to shift away from delivering directives as questions. Notice the difference between "Put your shoes on, please" and "Can you put on your shoes?" or even weaker, "Do you want to put on your shoes?" Sometimes people ask children questions that are meant to be commands but are taken literally by the children. In a case example, a child was asked "Do you want to leave the room to speak with the principal or stay here and listen?" The teacher expected the child to behave, as in her view being sent to the principal was a penalty. The child promptly got up and happily skipped off to the main office, taking the opportunity that was presented!

One way to reduce ineffective directives is to help parents pick tasks that they can monitor and control. If children learn that they can repeatedly ignore requests, it reduces the parents' authority. This may mean temporarily letting go of commands that cannot be enforced or increasing monitoring if the task is important.

When EB was 13, there was an opportunity to join a local tennis team, which her father wanted her to do. EB had no intention of going to the tennis practice, though she unconvincingly agreed to do so, assuming that her father would go to work and she would be responsible for taking the subway there herself. Once her father realized that she did not intend to go, as she had done with other activities, he increased monitoring to make sure she went and tried it. On the morning of the practice, instead of going to work, without forewarning or confrontation, he took her to practice. In this example, once she tried the activity and enjoyed it, he never had to miss work again to gain compliance.

Effective Communication Strategies to Support Behavioral Interventions

Feedback, shared agreements, limits, and rules rely on strong communication. Communicating goes beyond words; much is expressed with tone, touch, and body language. Help parents to build positive patterns in messaging and avoid communicating in ways that undermine their own strategies.

Command Doses

Medications are not the only treatments that come in doses. Think about interventions and communications in terms of doses, which are important to administer and mete out in the right amount. When parents give commands to children in a quiet and sweet tone of voice, the dose can be considered low. There are ways to increase the dose of a command, including by speaking loudly, making eye contact, using serious facial expressions, standing close to the child, and using physical touch. Caregivers can learn to recognize more potent ways to convey messages to their children.

However, a bigger dose of a command may not always be better. Yelling, which is a high-dose command, has a downside for both the parent and child in terms of modeling poor mood regulation, increasing conflict, and causing emotional upset. Yelling often follows when children have not responded to low-dose messages, leading parents to become frustrated. Sometimes children hear their parents' directives as "Maybe, maybe, NOW!" as opposed to "Please do X." Yelling, if done rarely, can have a bigger impact because it can startle a child who may be in danger, such as when walking in front of a moving vehicle. However, it may also have surprising results when the child does not expect it. When JDS's daughter was a toddler, she did not want to get in her car seat. JDS, who did not typically yell, decided to intentionally experiment with raising her voice to see if it would increase her daughter's willingness to comply. Though JDS expected greater volume to increase compliance, her daughter instead laughed, which was not the desired result. In this kind of situation, there will need to be experimentation and adjustments with the parents you coach when the intervention does not work as intended or expected.

Praise

It is important for parents to notice when children behave well. Praise and positive feedback, like commands, also come in doses. Some children need heavy doses of praise for it to penetrate. When children can absorb praise, there is great power in an adult beaming praise and a child taking it in completely.

However, though many children benefit from positive attention, other children are overwhelmed by it. These children struggle with hearing positive feedback, particularly if it is made with eye contact or a wide smile, suggesting that lower doses would be more effective for them. Some of the ways children show their discomfort in absorbing praise include looking away, becoming uncomfortable or upset, grunting, refuting it, or responding nastily. Parents can begin to read their children's cues to change the way praise is given so that it can be taken in. If children need a lower dose of praise, parents can shift to less eye contact, more muted tones, and more banal content, such as "That worked okay," as opposed to "FANTASTIC JOB!" Another way to reduce the dose is to tell the child indirectly by saying to someone else in earshot: "You know, Janey picked up her room today."

Praise is better accepted when it is focal, specific, and genuine, and the basis for it is within the person's control (Barkley, 2013; Kazdin, 2008). When adults "lay on" praise that is false or exaggerated, it can have the opposite effect than intended and can be interpreted as sarcastic or disingenuous. Worksheets 10.1, "Ways to Praise Your Child," and 10.2, "How Does My Child Take In Praise?," found at the end of the chapter, can help you work with parents on how to deliver praise and recognize how their child responds.

Feedback

One of your jobs in helping parents is to identify ways for them to provide effective feedback to their children. Remember that feedback can be both verbal and nonverbal. Think about the value of a warm touch, a knowing look, a hug, or a bright smile for the child who appreciates it. Interpersonal reinforcement has no financial cost and is very powerful. Similarly, a scowl or dour look can have an equally powerful effect. In addition, optimal feedback from parents does not make love conditional ("I love you when . . ." or "I love you if . . ."). Children will notice the conditionality of love and warmth, whether deliberately meant or not.

Feedback also works well when the parent and the child are on the same page about the targeted behavior. Up through third grade, EB's daughter was very careful about her attire, and especially enjoyed wearing dresses. In fourth grade her style changed. However, one day, she came to breakfast looking neater than usual for that school year. EB said, "You look nice today." With sincerity, her daughter responded, "Thanks, Mom. I'll change." For her daughter, the feedback was useful in that her intended aim was not to look nice. This certainly was not EB's aim in providing the feedback.

"Catch Them When They're Good"

It is easy to notice when children do not behave as we would like. Parents notice and comment on those instances. Many caregivers do not also notice and acknowledge when their child is doing something well, helpful, useful, or prosocial. Their children, though, likely do notice the differential feedback they get from their caregivers. The times when parents fail to notice their child doing something nice, helpful, or well are often missed opportunities. Parents may feel that these behaviors are expected and, therefore, not worthy of comment. A child doing expected chores or self-care without a fuss may be an opportunity for positive comments. Not bothering a sibling, allowing a parent to talk on the phone without interruption, and responding to interactions positively may all be worthy of recognition, depending upon the child.

"Catch them when they're good" is a helpful mantra for parents to use to cue themselves to give positive feedback. We are not sure who coined this phrase, but it highlights the importance of shifting the feedback stream to the child's good behavior. When there is more positivity from parents, children tend to be more upbeat as well. It does require the child to do something for the parent to catch and the parent has to be able to notice. Some parent training programs offer easier commands, such as Barkley's (2013) "fetch commands," in order to increase the opportunity for praising the child's compliant behavior. These are small, easy commands that the child is highly likely to follow, providing an almost guaranteed opportunity for praise. An example might be "Please grab me a tissue."

Some caregivers need help brainstorming situations when they can catch their child being good. They struggle to think of times that their child behaves in a manner worthy of positive feedback. They may think that the behavior has to be significant to deserve such a response. Talk through possibilities and opportunities for them to provide praise and give the caregiver a variety of ways to commend their child.

5:1 Ratio

Kazdin (2008) recommends that families strive to provide five times as many positive feedback communications as critiques. Many parents find this assignment difficult, but also eye-opening. Often in reactive households the ratio of positive statements made to children as compared with negative statements is reversed from the desired 5:1 ratio, and the bulk of the feedback is negative. Sadly, some children believe, based on the amount of negative feedback, that their parents do not like them or would be better off without them. Given the high stakes of these beliefs, it is a worthwhile pattern to alter.

When it is difficult to get parents to provide the 5:1 ratio, another suggestion to give parents as homework can be to tell their child at night one thing that they did well during that day. It is startling how many caregivers report that they cannot identify one good behavior. Parents may need help in identifying the proverbial needle in the haystack. When you help parents script these daily messages, you also enable them to do the following: reduce the anger, signal that the parent has forgiven the child, instill hope for the future, and notice when skills are being developed. When the parent is finding it difficult to identify something positive in the child's behavior try suggesting these comments:

"You got into bed even though it was hard for you."
"I noticed you playing with your LEGOs when you were sad."
"I know you were mad, but I'm glad you told me."
"I heard from your teacher that . . . "
"You calmed down a little faster than usual. How'd you do that?"
"You had a tough day. I'm sure we can make tomorrow better."
"We'll try again tomorrow. I love you"

Worksheet 10.3, "Exploring When Things Went Well," helps a caregiver identify times when their child did behave well and what might have helped that happen.

Acknowledgment versus Praise

Despite the seeming appeal of increasing parental praise, Marshall (2010) recommends shifting from prizes and praise to acknowledgement, because it allows the child to own their successes, rather than making changes to please their parents. Similarly, Kohn (1993) addresses the risks of decreasing intrinsic motivation by encouraging children to engage in certain behaviors to please others rather than themselves. When teaching parents the subtleties of providing positive feedback, there is value in learning the skill of acknowledgement: "I notice you are making your bed," as opposed to "Thank you for making your bed so nicely for me."

Consistency and Expectations: Recognizing Patterns and Developing Positive Ones

Children and their parents should have a general sense of how the day will unfold, what will be allowed, what works, and how typical situations will be addressed. Ideally the daily patterns that develop are understandable, intentional, flexible, and work toward everyone's best interest.

Surprisingly, sometimes children and parents do not recognize patterns. For example, after every session a child patient demanded that her mother buy her ice cream. When asked if her mother was likely to say yes, she seemed to believe she would, although her mother had said no every time before. Parents can have a similar "blindness" about how their children are likely to respond. When there is a clear pattern, help parents identify their expectations for behavior and rules, plan their own responses, implement the plan consistently, evaluate the success of their responses, and fine-tune expectations as needed. Help both parents and children become aware of and change their strategies to increase interpersonal effectiveness. In the ice cream situation, the therapist worked with the child to identify the pattern and plan a new way to engage. In her case, she switched to "When can I have ice cream?" The child was able to consider the benefits of waiting (delay of gratification) and communicating in a way that would more likely yield a parental yes.

Building on Success

When a child has a successful experience, especially in an identified developmental challenge area (becoming toilet trained, reading, riding a bike, driving a car), it creates momentum and enthusiasm for continued effort. By achieving repeated small goals children feel good about themselves and are less likely to be dysregulated. Conversely, repeated frustration and failure lead to difficulty in feeling good about anything, which is a reason for focusing therapy on creating small accomplishments.

We are trying to build both success and feelings of success in children and caregivers who have not had positive experiences in their interactions. This chapter focused on a number of ways to create positive interactions, develop confidence and functional communication in family members, and shift the tenor of the parent–child relationship.

WORKSHEET 10.1

Ways to Praise Your Child

Low dose:

- A quiet look or smile
- Telling another adult about the child's accomplishment with child at a distance
- Touching the child's shoulder
- Hanging up a picture the child drew
- "I noticed that you . . ."
- A quiet "thanks"

Medium dose:

- A high five
- "Thank you for . . ." (with more energy)
- A brighter smile and a positive look
- A direct comment on the child's accomplishment

High dose:

- Big smile!
- Big hug!
- Beaming positive attention and enthusiastic comment
- "You're really good at . . ."
- "That was really helpful . . ."
- Tell other people, with the child next to you, what you appreciated.

WORKSHEET 10.2

How Does My Child Take In Praise?

People receive praise differently. We want praise to be useful. Figuring out how your child takes in praise will help you deliver it effectively.

- How do you typically like to give praise?
- How does your child receive praise?
- What dose of praise works for your child?
- What makes it more likely that your child will respond well and take praise in (e.g., eye contact, accompanying touch, a high five, praise that is not too over the top)?
- How can you tell that your child heard the praise and responded well?
- What is the dosage of praise that works well with your child?
- Do you want to be giving more praise, less praise, or the same amount of praise as you have been giving?
- Is there a match or mismatch between how you offer praise and how your child receives it? If so, what can bring those two things closer together?

Notes:

WORKSHEET 10.3

Exploring When Things Went Well

- What went well?

- How could I tell?

- How did I feel?

- How did my child seem to feel? How could I tell?

- What seemed to help?

- How did I enjoy the moment?

CHAPTER 11

Monitoring Behavior as an Intervention

The process of monitoring, or paying attention to behaviors, can have both benefits and risks (Nassau et al., 2009). There is value in keeping track of behaviors to get a baseline on a phenomenon and find out if an intervention changes it. For example, facilitating the 5:1 ratio, as described in the previous chapter, requires parents to monitor both their child's behavior in order to find opportunities for praise and their own behavior in order to keep track of how often they take those opportunities. Monitoring can improve behaviors that a family wishes to change (Compernolle et al., 2019), but it is not a neutral activity. Use monitoring with care, because attending to some behaviors has the potential to worsen the outcome, as in over-attending to pain (Kohl et al., 2013) or overfocusing on negative behaviors.

Monitoring the Child's Behavior

Keeping Track

When you talk to parents about monitoring behavior, be specific about how to do it. We often ask caregivers to keep track of "ABCs"—meaning antecedents, behavior, and consequences—in order to detect patterns or gather baseline data against which we can compare change. This is not intended to be an opportunity for parents to complain in session about the child's difficult behavior from the week.

For example, a therapist was seeing a mother for parent guidance regarding her son. The mother enthusiastically left a session with homework that involved monitoring her son's challenging behaviors to get baseline data to see whether she and the therapist could detect patterns. In the next session she began listing every difficult behavior her son had exhibited over the prior week, both large and small. She did not also talk about what he had done well. The therapist, taken by surprise, did not have a chance to redirect her. Unfortunately, her son was in the office for some of the session and wound up yelling in the office and stating that he hated coming to therapy. This monitoring did not serve the intended purpose. Monitoring a child's behavior to make a case about their "badness" will lead the child to feel worse about themselves. In addition, when a child is in the midst of a meltdown, attempting to monitor their behavior by video, audio, or even by writing down what occurred, often escalates the situation. Instead caregivers can, later on when they are alone, note the basic information about the situation.

In a parent's retelling of their children's problematic behavior, they are more likely to describe the child's behavior than their own because the child's behavior is what they want to change. Another reason they might not describe their own behavior is because they are embarrassed, whether they view themselves as too harsh, too permissive, or too enabling of the negative behavior pattern. In order to get this important piece of the puzzle, alleviate the parent's discomfort in describing their own behavior by being nonjudgmental by reminding them that this is what you hope to help with and by letting them know that you have experience with many families struggling with similar problems. You and they may discover something in their actions that is inadvertently maintaining or reinforcing their child's difficult behavior.

Suggest that parents measure specific target behaviors. Keep it manageable, noting the date, day of the week, the time, and what was happening before, during, and after the behavior occurred. Keep it short, but with enough detail to discern patterns.

CASE STUDY: Identifying the Usual Suspects

Spencer's parents sought parent guidance because Spencer had tantrums almost every day. His parents did not understand why and did not see any patterns in what they or he was doing. He was often a happy child without other notable difficult behaviors. His parents had not found effective ways to deescalate his tantrums: Instead, they let them run their course. Their therapist suggested that they track some details about when the tantrums happened, what was going on at the time, and what occurred afterward. In doing so, they noticed that the tantrums tended to happen on weekday afternoons, with little apparent provocation. Spencer would take umbrage with something his parent or younger sibling said and would start escalating. He would initially be sassy and then, when he was told that his tone of voice was not appropriate, he would begin to yell and continue yelling until he stormed out of the room to his bedroom, slamming the door. His parents did not like the door slamming and would scold him, which led to more yelling. The therapist asked what was Spencer's routine when he returned home from school, and his parents noted that there was no clear routine. They usually asked him to do his homework, but that was about it.

Thinking about the usual suspects, the therapist asked when lunch was served at school. The family realized that lunch was served very early and that Spencer probably came home hungry every day. Further, in other situations, Spencer often had difficulty with transitions, but did well with a set routine when one was established. The parents monitored what they did upon his return from school as well. They realized that when they were reunited with Spencer after a school day or a playdate, they asked him many questions about his time away.

With the help of the parent guidance expert, the parents implemented a new routine, in which a snack was waiting for Spencer on the table when he got home from school. They created a visual chart of what Spencer was to do when he came home. It showed that he took off his backpack and coat, sat down, had his snack, decided whether he would take a 30-minute break to listen to music or watch television, and then get out his homework. The parents also stopped peppering him with questions. Instead, they decided to talk about their "roses and thorns" at dinner. Each family member would mention something they enjoyed about the day and something they wished did not happen. Once Spencer was provided with an afterschool snack and had a more predictable routine, the tantrums disappeared.

Worksheets 11.1, "Behavior Detective: Part I," and 11.2, "Behavior Detective: Part II," are useful for monitoring behavior, detecting patterns, and determining relevant aspects of the situation.

Why Does This Behavior Continue?

This section focuses on using the PACT model to manage difficult behaviors when they occur, to reduce their impact, and to prevent a host of other challenges through more careful assessment of behavior, choosing which intervention to use, and treating the problem (implement the intervention).

Get to the Root of the Problem

As part of your parent guidance assessment (the "A" in "PACT"), you will be thinking about not only what the problem is, but what maintains it and underlies it. Monitoring, as described previously, will help. There are common triggers for children that you can ask about, such as "No," "You can't," "You need to be finished with that," or "You have to." Some interventions, such as collaborative problem solving, later developed into collaborative and proactive solutions, or CPS (Greene, 1998, 2016), contain mechanisms for getting to the root of the problem. Greene's Plan B, which is an essential CPS tool, requires parents to spend time understanding the child's perspective and to explain their own as well before trying to solve the problem. Take the following example of a child not wanting to take a shower:

- *Step 1: Empathy:* "You don't want to take a shower. How come?" This concern is then explored with the child.
- *Step 2: Parent's concern:* "I worry that kids will tease you when you smell" (or whatever their concern is).
- *Step 3: Problem solving:* "What can we do about it?"

It is useful to have a detailed understanding of the nature of the problem before trying to solve it. In another example, the parents of a usually cooperative fifth grader came for parent guidance. They were angry with the daughter and had punished her by taking away her screen time, but she was still engaging in the negative behavior.

Each night they told her to come in from playing in the neighborhood at 5:00 P.M. She was predictably late every night and had consistently lost her evening screen time as a result. The parents shifted to using Plan B. They started with: "You are home after five o'clock every night. What's up?" She answered, "I don't know what time it is." The parents purchased her a wristwatch, because they felt she was too young for a cell phone, and she consistently came home on time after she began wearing it. In this case, they did not have to come to a solution together. The strategy of exploring what was behind their daughter's behavior helped them better understand the reason for it.

Is the Child's Behavior Reasonable?

Sometimes parents wish their child would behave differently even when there may be no reasonable way for the child to do so in the particular circumstance. If you cannot reasonably answer the question "What would have been a better coping choice?" then maybe the behavior should not be seen as misbehavior. In a case example, the parents had set a goal for a child to get along with his older sibling in the morning. He would not have access to his Nintendo games until he had 2 consecutive days without a problem. The dilemma was that his sibling instigated battles all morning. When asked, "Is it possible for anyone to get along with her in the morning?" the parents reported that it was in fact not possible.

Does the Child Have the Requisite Skills for Success?

Many times children do not have the necessary skills to succeed with regard to behavioral expectations. Assessing the child's ability to meet expectations is essential. For example, a school meeting was arranged for a "misbehaving" middle school student. The school staff were frustrated with the student because every time they asked him to work on math he refused. When the young teenager at the meeting was asked, "Why aren't you doing the work?" he replied, "I can't do it." The school team then asked him why he did not say that he had this problem before, and he responded, "I used to say "I can't,' but then the teachers said, 'Yes, you can.'" The teen's math skills were later assessed, and he was found to actually have a learning disability in the subject.

Children typically do not want to get in trouble and there are many reasons why a child might not be able to behave. They may have low frustration tolerance and need to develop the ability to tolerate frustration first. They may be more impulsive than the average child their age. They may be particularly susceptible to becoming "hangry" (irritable when hungry). There are many other possibilities as well.

Is the Behavior Secondary to a Different Diagnosis?

In thinking about behavior, if the "why" is not assessed, underlying problems and diagnoses can be missed. When motivational strategies are not working, question why they are not and whether the target of the intervention should change.

Consider the parents of a 10-year-old boy who were frustrated by his refusal to brush his teeth. In a session with the therapist, the parents announced their plan to make him stay in the bathroom the night of the appointment until he brushed his teeth. The parent guidance expert asked at the next session whether that plan had worked. The parents reported that they gave up at 3:00 A.M. The child reported after the parents left the room: "Oh, I've got to teach them that's not going to work." Realizing that forced bathroom time would not solve the problem, the parents followed up on the therapist's recommendation to pursue sensory integration treatment through occupational therapy (OT). Even though the boy was strong-willed, he did have an issue with oral sensitivity and, with the assistance of an OT, he was able to tolerate toothbrushing. His behavior appeared to be oppositionality and a battle of wills; however, these problems were secondary to his sensory sensitivity.

Is the Goal Behavior Doable for the Child?

Some parents need help in identifying what their children are actually capable of doing. Part of your job as a parent guidance consultant is to assist caregivers in understanding child development and their child, so that they can challenge their children to learn new skills without generating impossible tasks. What is doable? What is never doable? What might be doable under unique circumstances but is frustratingly difficult?

Help parents keep challenges in the doable range. Habits and patterns of behavior can be difficult to change, so we want them trending in positive directions. When thinking of the challenges to behave well, remember that not only is the difficulty of the task at issue, but also when the task is happening and the child's stamina for ongoing challenges. Remind parents that a situation not going well does not mean that all progress is lost. Progress is rarely linear when people seek to change, with no return to problem behavior or emotions. All is not lost when some difficulty arises.

Does the Child's Negative Behavior Work?

Challenging behavior may succeed in getting children what they are seeking. When asked directly, some children explicitly say, "I get what I want when I beg [or scream or cry]." The end of a difficult interaction may inadvertently be rewarding to the child. But it is often more subtle than this case indicates, as shown in the next two examples.

Parents report to you that their teenage daughter is on her phone with friends until late in the evening. She does not start her homework until 9:30 P.M. and is up until very late completing it. When asked by the therapist why she does not do her homework and then call her friends, she replied "If I finished my homework at 10:00 P.M., my parents wouldn't let me stay up to talk to friends, but they would let me stay up to finish my homework." She had figured out that reversing the order would not work in helping her to achieve her goal of social time with friends.

When asked to clean his room, a teenage boy would run away and start slamming the glass door in the family's home. The parents were terrified that the glass would shatter and hurt a family member. He was asked by his therapist why he chose the glass door and not the closer wooden doors. He replied that his parents only stopped making requests when he slammed the more dangerous door. These examples demonstrate that children can have effective, though perhaps not healthy or helpful, behavioral plans that they utilize on their parents.

Does the Child Understand Expectations?

Decipher whether children knowingly made a mistake or really did not understand the rules of behavior. If penalties for negative behavior are going to be imposed by parents, make certain that the child intentionally misbehaved. Consider the first grader on the playground with peers. He had a mild cold, which led to coughing and spitting. Another child came close to him. He immediately warned her to move away as he was going to spit. When she did not move away, he spit at her, believing that he was justified in doing so since he gave her a warning. He seemed puzzled by his mother's demand that he apologize. Only in a postgame conversation did he understand that spitting, particularly at people, is perceived as very problematic, just as hitting someone would be. Once the child received this explanation, this behavior did not recur.

Monitoring Parents' Behavior

Self-monitoring for caregivers helps identify their patterns of behavior and emotions, vulnerabilities or triggers, and unhelpful patterns of responding. It allows for understanding what behaviors they would like to change and for keeping track of what they feel are positive changes, as they implement interventions. Monitoring specific parental behaviors, such as the use of praise and criticism, can help guide parent coaching. For example, parent–child interaction therapy (PCIT; Funderburk & Eyberg, 2011) specifically monitors behaviors in parents in order to work toward certain benchmarks, such as reducing criticism, sarcasm, and other negative responses to the child.

Identify specific and discrete behaviors to monitor. You are more likely to attain good data if you are clear about what you want parents to keep track of. For example, you might say, "Could you use your phone or a notepad to write down every time you say something positive to your child?" Alternatively, you might ask a caregiver to, at the end of the day, write down what interactions with their child got them angry and how they responded.

CASE STUDY: The Benefit of Data

Alisha and her parent guidance therapist had talked a lot about how arguments with her granddaughter escalated. Alisha reported that it usually started with her granddaughter being "on edge." The therapist asked her to keep track of what happened, particularly how Alisha responded when her granddaughter was starting to escalate. At the next session she brought in a log of four arguments that had taken place during the week. As the therapist looked at the logs with her, they noticed that

Alisha was not following the agreed-upon plan to listen and empathize with her granddaughter before starting to make suggestions. Instead, Alisha tried to be helpful by heading right into her own suggestions, which caused her granddaughter to escalate, and left Alisha feeling hurt and resentful when her granddaughter rejected her help. She and the therapist identified the barriers to starting with validation. They practiced and role played validating and withholding suggestions. The next week went much more smoothly for both Alisha and her granddaughter. It was also surprising to Alisha that when she listened first, her granddaughter seemed to accept many more of her suggestions.

Monitoring is a useful practice for caregivers that has multiple benefits, including making parents more aware of what they and their child are doing. It is useful to have the data in order to monitor progress and develop appropriate behavioral intervention plans. The next chapter provides strategies for implementing motivational systems.

WORKSHEET 11.1

Behavior Detective: Part I

Jot down the circumstances around instances of the target behavior or when the target behavior was predicted to happen but did not.

What happened and with whom?	Where?	Time of day	Date and day of week	Outcomes and reactions (in the environment and from other people)	Things that made it harder or easier to manage

WORKSHEET 11.2

Behavior Detective: Part II

When do things go well?

___

___

___

When do things go poorly?

___

___

___

What are some patterns I see? Can I make any predictions?

___

___

___

What are all of the choices for making it better even if I don't want to choose them?

___

___

___

What can I try in the future?

___

___

___

Notes for achieving success:

___

___

___

CHAPTER 12

Working with Motivational Systems

Alexandra was a student in a kindergarten classroom that utilized a whole-class reward system. Each day the students had two opportunities to earn a sticker. When a child earned nine stickers, they could pick a prize that was special for having earned it rather than for any real enjoyment value. Stickers could be obtained in two ways: either by helping clean up after the morning free-play activity or by resting well during the class quiet time. The second opportunity was confusing because the children rated themselves. Students were asked if they had done well during the rest time, which they signaled with a thumbs-up or thumbs-down. There were no clear guidelines about what constituted "doing well." Sometimes the teacher disagreed with the child's assessment, both denying them the sticker and adding punishing embarrassment for having rated themselves more positively than they deserved. On the day before Alexandra's fifth birthday, she announced to her parents that she had earned eight of the stickers and was certain, given her track record of earning every sticker, to obtain one of the prizes on her actual birthday.

Unfortunately, Alexandra was taken out of class for a school hearing screening at cleanup time and was, therefore, denied the opportunity to earn the first sticker. After class quiet time, her teacher asked her if she had done well and Alexandra, fearful of embarrassment and overwhelmed by the enormity of the moment, hesitated before giving the thumbs-up, and this sticker was also denied. She became distressed, an unexpected side effect of participating in an unnecessary program, because Alexandra tended to be cooperative in school without additional reward. Furthermore, she believed the penalty was for unknowingly doing something wrong during rest time, as the parameters for doing well were ill defined. She did not understand that the penalty was for her hesitation. When people do not know what they have done wrong, it impairs their ability to improve their behavior going forward.

Effective Use of Behavioral Systems

Reward charts can go wrong in many ways. It is important to remember that what can help can hurt as well. The previous example shows the importance of careful design when implementing a behavioral program. This teacher would have done well to remember the acronym "SMART" to set her class goals: "specific, measurable, achievable, relevant, and timely" (Doran, 1981). Did the classroom reward system meet those requirements? In some ways it did. It was specific, though not clear, timely, measurable, or achievable for most students. The lack of clarity caused implementation trouble for Alexandra. Did it serve to improve anyone's rest time or cleanup behavior? The target behaviors were unimportant or irrelevant for most, if not all, of the children in the class, who had already established these behaviors without requiring a reward. For the children with impulse control difficulties and other behavioral problems, their issues did not revolve around cleanup. Though these children did often have trouble resting, the reward system was not powerful or targeted appropriately to bring about the desired change.

Seemingly unintentionally, the second sticker required more than good rest-time behavior; it also demanded the ability to reflect on that behavior and manage social anxiety. The teacher seemed perplexed that, with good rest-time behavior, Alexandra hesitated to give the "thumbs- up." She felt that she needed to punish her hesitation because it was "a behavior," meaning that it was both unwanted and intentional. Everything is a behavior. The useful question to ask is what does that behavior signify? In this chapter, we discuss techniques to target behaviors most effectively as well as help parents develop and implement behavioral systems.

A Quick Primer on Behaviorism

Many behavioral terms are used by the general population, often incorrectly, leading to confusion. We cannot review all the intricacies of behavioral principles—the subject of many books—but we cover the details that you need to know in order to convey them to parents. Scott et al. (2023) review some of these concepts.

- A consequence is what happens following a behavior.
- A reinforcer increases a behavior in frequency or intensity. Giving a child a cookie when they say "please" is a reinforcer. Sometimes parents do something that seems likely to reduce a behavior, such as yelling, but it actually provides attention that acts as a reinforcer, thereby increasing the behavior. Reinforcement is about increasing behavior, whether intentional or not.
- Punishments reduce behavior.
- Positive reinforcement occurs when something is added in order to increase a behavior. In behaviorism, the word *positive* denotes adding something into the system and the word *negative* indicates removing something. Some common examples of positive reinforcement are praise and prizes following desired behaviors.
- Negative reinforcement is not punishment. It is taking something aversive away in order to increase behavior. An example of negative reinforcement would be

lecturing a teenager on washing their face. In order to avoid the time-consuming parent lecture ("All right already, I'll do it"), the teenager complies. Another example is taking a pain reliever to respond to a headache (aversive stimulus). If the headache goes away, then the person is more likely to take the pain reliever again in the future. If the headache does not go away, then the medication-taking behavior was not reinforced.

- Similarly, positive punishment is adding something to reduce a behavior. An example of positive punishment is assigning additional homework when the class behaves poorly. Since students do not typically like more work (unpleasant), adding (positive) will reduce the poor behavior (punishment).
- Negative punishment involves removing something in order to reduce a behavior. If a child misbehaves and, as a result, is not allowed to watch television, the removal of television is the negative punishment if it works as intended. Grounding is another common parental use of negative punishment, since the parent is removing the fun of being out with friends.
- Extinction is a strategy of withdrawing the response to a behavior so that, without reinforcement, the behavior will fade. For example, if parents ignore whining, thus rendering it ineffective for getting attention or giving in to what the child is whining about, they hope that the child will no longer whine. If parents use this strategy, they need to know that there can be an "extinction burst" during which the behavior actually increases (the burst) before it fades in the absence of reinforcement. Caregivers should also know that if they respond at all, even after a long absence of response, the response can serve to increase the persistence of a behavior. If reinforcement is unpredictable, it can unintentionally reinforce the behavior more powerfully than if the ignoring had never occurred.

It is not useful, and may worsen the situation, to punish or offer a child rewards for behaviors that are out of the range of the child's skill set. It is equally unhelpful to utilize consequences that do not appreciate the full picture of why people do what they do. The Public Broadcasting Service (PBS) produced a powerful documentary (*The Trouble with Evan*, Frontline, 1994) highlighting this error. Evan, age 11 (an actual patient and not an actor), engages in many problematic behaviors, including lying, stealing, and defying his parents. Evan and his parents receive therapy and parent guidance to improve his behavior. With footage from their therapy and home videos, the viewer soon learns the punch line, that the trouble with Evan is really the environment in which he is living. The documentary exposes the dangers in implementing ineffective and superficial interventions, such as advising Evan to "try harder" by doing chores at home.

Motivational systems (such as sticker charts) can be designed with parents to effectively increase and decrease behaviors. The marking of the behavior on a chart builds in accountability for both parents and children in committing to a structured course of action and recognizing what improvement would look like. In the sections that follow we discuss ways to boost the effectiveness of this intervention when it is carefully chosen and systematized.

Many parents and therapists overuse sticker charts as their primary go-to intervention for child behavior problems. When programs are hastily developed, they can fail because the creators neglect to take into account differing motivations, causes of behavior, and what is achievable by the particular child. An example of a common behavior for parents to target is getting ready for school in the morning. Although parents are often highly motivated to get their children to school on time, children may prefer to get there as late as possible, if not skip school entirely! Identifying these motivations can assist in developing more organic solutions, such as getting to school early enough to have time in the playground with a preferred peer, which may be more motivating to the child than just the prospect of another school day. Consider motivations and environmental factors before choosing how to target behavior.

Prioritizing Behaviors to Target

When designing a behavioral system, a good place to start is by identifying the important behaviors that the parents would like to address first. When there is more than one targeted behavior, choose what to focus on initially. Factors to consider in choosing a starting point may include the seriousness of the behavior, the child's motivation to fix it, the ease of fixing it, the frequency of the behavior, and the ability to measure and observe the behavior. Parents are sometimes disappointed that not everything can be addressed at once, but you can reassure them that tabled behaviors can be the focus of intervention at a later date. Employ the concept of "yet." "They don't have good table manners yet" is more hopeful than "They don't have good table manners." Success with behavioral plans depends on helping the caregiver in making the behavior and expectation clear, not targeting too many things at one time, focusing on the first step of a solution (not too big a jump), and choosing either important or easier problems to solve initially.

Sometimes caregivers focus on what we consider less-important behavior. Parents may be particularly bothered by issues such as poor table manners, even when other behaviors like aggression toward siblings, which we may prioritize, are occurring simultaneously. Another example we have seen is parents who are focusing on the child's tone when the child's message may be a more important concern. A stark example is the teen who yells, "I'm going to kill myself," provoking the parent to yell back, "Stop yelling at me," rather than focusing on the important message. That said, parents are people too and sometimes center on their own feelings rather than on the child's immediate message. As therapists, we can work to understand the issues that tend to be more important to parents than to some of us, such as manners, cursing, lying, and tone of voice. Step one may be to carefully think through the priorities of the family when introducing any behavioral plan.

Caregivers also benefit from education from us about making behavioral system choices, breaking them down into doable steps, and looking at the underlying factors that drive negative behavior. Doable is key to a functional system. We want the children to earn the rewards; otherwise they are useless.

When parents achieve early success with behavioral intervention, they become excited and sometimes try to add in all of the behaviors they wish to change simultaneously. A singular, focused approach, in which one skill or behavior at a time is addressed, is usually superior. EB uses the analogy of a tennis lesson. When she takes an hour-long tennis lesson, there is too much feedback for her to absorb. It is difficult to prioritize what to fix, and sometimes the suggestions blend together and are lost. A 30-minute lesson yields fewer suggestions for change and worked better for her.

The less-is-more approach to feedback can be more useful in many situations. This was the case with an aggressive 8-year-old girl whose parents devised a specific program to reduce hitting with the help of their parent guidance therapist. In 2 weeks, she went from more than 30 episodes of hitting to 2 minor incidents. The parents were delighted and without consulting with the therapist they changed the program before their next session to include all of the girl's negative comments, her cursing, and her throwing behavior (which occurred many times an hour) as targets of change. The child was not able to be successful with this new plan, nor were the parents able to monitor all of the behaviors. None of these behaviors improved, and the hitting returned to its baseline. After the unsuccessful expansion of the behavioral plan, it was much harder to reinstate the original successful program than it had been to introduce it in the first place.

Constructing Reward Programs

Parents use immediate rewards frequently, even if they are unaware that they are doing so. "If you leave the park, we can get ice cream." or "If you finish your homework, we'll go to the toy store." are typical examples. Some parents are also familiar with more sophisticated reward charts and systems, especially around toilet training and hygiene. Kazdin (2008) has a systematic way to develop reward programs so that children earn a prize after a short interval, with longer term, more meaningful rewards earned after sustained desired behavior. In Kazdin's (2008) program, children earn a small prize quickly, which helps them feel hopeful about achieving their goals. He uses the harder-to-earn reward in order to motivate children who benefit from a more substantial marker of their success. An example might be a child makes their bed five times and gets to play a game with their parents. After 3 months of making their bed, the child earns a trip to a water park.

Choose specific, measurable focal behaviors that the child is capable of achieving and set an appropriate interval of time in which to earn the reinforcer. By capable, we intend for target behaviors to require some additional effort, but not so much support that the child will not regularly be able to succeed. At the start the prize should be earned fairly quickly, so that the child becomes hopeful about behavior change and trusts that they will receive the agreed-upon rewards. Requiring consecutive units (hours or days) of successful behavior can be problematic when children can lose all the progress they have made after one mistake. Early prizes should be interesting enough to motivate the child but not so big that they cannot be replicated or lead to the child refusing to engage in the same behavior in the future for a more reasonable reward. Additionally, huge rewards signal a higher task difficulty, whereas we want the parent to signal that a behavior is manageable. Younger children, or those who have difficulty delaying gratification, may need a more immediate reward in order to understand and follow the program.

Let parents know that one side effect of reward systems is that they can create problematic barter systems in families. When parents give prizes frequently, or suggest payment for everyday behaviors, children can start to behave as disgruntled employees when asked to do any activities for the family. Rather than doing tasks because they are a member of the family, children might begin to do them only for a reward. Building in reciprocity and helpfulness without payment at an early age is also a useful value. If children develop a bartering mentality, they are likely to respond to commands, with the refrain "What will you give me if I . . . ?" rather than having a sense that they are a citizen of the household and, as such, they need to help make the household function. If this dynamic becomes a regular and ongoing concern, then behavioral programs must be adjusted.

When devising a behavioral program for the parents with whom you work, be very careful to avoid programs that pit siblings against each other. Families often believe that healthy competition will improve motivation. Although it can, it can also foster conflict. Programs can often be cooperative, benefiting each of the siblings when they do well, or have an element that makes it positive for both of them when one does well, such as playing a fun game, or a cooperative activity, like an escape room. It is also important to avoid incentivizing other children in the family to misbehave in order to then be able to earn rewards.

Worksheet 12.1, "Developing a Behavior Plan," reviews some questions to ask to help caregivers think through how to effectively develop a behavioral program.

Helping Parents Choose Rewards

When possible, help parents choose rewards that develop other skills or are positive and doable for the family. Interpersonal rewards such as high fives, hugs, praise, or a game together can be very positive and motivating. Just as parents should not pick punishments that punish themselves more, they should not pick rewards that punish themselves either. If parents do not believe in a particular prize (weapons, devices, ear piercing, Barbies), using them as rewards does not make sense. Poor choice of reward will lead to more difficulties down the line when the parent is not comfortable with the child receiving the prize they earned. Sometimes parents, who are uncomfortable with a prize, set the target so high that the child cannot achieve it, thereby sabotaging the system. We have seen this outcome with rewards involving money, unrealistic pets, trips, and cars. This practice builds hopelessness and a lack of trust between parents and children. Parents should feel comfortable giving a prize, preferably one that is already on hand, when it is earned.

Part of devising the system with parents is choosing these reasonable reward targets. Consider the nature of the rewards with the caveats we discuss in mind. While some rewards can build family bonding, such as earning something to share with siblings, others are problematic. Depending upon how they are designed, food prizes might lead to unhealthy feelings about treats. Earning money is controversial, even if a prize would be more expensive than the payment provided. We have seen this reward used effectively, but be judicious in its use. Receiving a pet, especially a family pet such as a dog or a cat, is also an ill-advised choice especially when maintaining good behavior is required to keep the pet and when the expectation is that the child will do all of the pet care. Most family activities, such as those involving food, and general routines should be noncontingent (not earned). If children benefit from engaging in sports, through which they can achieve success and use energy appropriately, these activities should also be noncontingent.

It can also be unwise to provide a reward that requires engaging in a negative behavior to earn it. For example, at the start of the school year, a kindergarten student was running and hiding under a table instead of engaging in her classroom activities. A reward system was devised by her school, in which she was required her to come out from under the table five times to earn stickers toward an ice cream sandwich. She started the program. It was immediately successful in some ways. She came out from under the table more quickly each time. The problem was that she was also hiding under the table more frequently than before the program was implemented. When asked why, she replied, "You don't get the sticker unless you come out from under the table." The program was altered to give a time-based reward for not going under the table at all, and the behavior immediately improved.

There are many prizes that do work. Choosing one depends upon the family and the child, with the caveats just discussed in mind. Stickers that can add up to larger prizes work for many children. Small toys or books that the child helps to choose are useful. A child might like to earn extra time with preferred activities, such as screen time, or with having their bedtime moved a little later on a particular night. Fun events, such as dinners out or a movie night, can work if the child is excited about them, and can also provide positive family time together. Special food rewards can work if they are not likely to cause other problems and there are no ongoing food issues. Brainstorm with the child and caregiver what the child might find motivating and what the parent feels is acceptable, doable, and an appropriate size for the effort and outcome.

Always Follow Through on Rewards

Encourage parents to be ready to deliver the prize, whatever it is, if the child earned it. We have both seen several children who were motivated to earn a reward, changed their behavior, and then did not receive it. When children do not receive the reward as promised, the behavior often reverts to its previous baseline and the child is less motivated to try again. Further, they learn that they cannot count on their parents to follow through on what they say they will do.

Other Ways to Shift Behavior

Build Incompatible Behavior

In thinking with parents about shifting child habits, one strategy is to replace undesirable habits with incompatible behaviors. This is frequently attempted by parents when a child hits a peer or pet and they try to replace the behavior with "touch nicely." The problem in this example is that often this replacement behavior gives the hitter easier access to hit the target again! A more effective incompatible behavior to reduce hitting might be to place hands together and wiggle thumbs up and down in circles or to press hands together and take three deep breaths. If a child frequently whines when asking for something, practicing smiling and saying "please" can be incompatible behaviors. With dogs, often the owners identify jumping and barking at guests as undesirable behaviors. Owners define the more positive behavior, sitting quietly in one spot, which is incompatible with barking and jumping.

Make It Easier to Engage in the Desirable Behavior

In addition to exchanging negative behaviors for more positive counterparts, another strategy for parents is to build behaviors intentionally, either by attaching new behaviors to existing habits or by defining the small shaping steps required to ultimately build a new sequence of behaviors. With a habit that works every day, such as toothbrushing, it may be easier to add a new habit to that one. For example, if a teenager is taking a new daily medication, place the pill bottle near the morning toothbrush or their charging cell phone.

Other habits and new skills may have to be taught in steps. Surprisingly, sometimes when teaching new behaviors, it is easier to start at the end and build the steps backward rather than forward, in a method known as backward chaining (Najdowski, 2017). When using this method, the parents help with the prior steps so that the child can achieve the final one, and then work backward. Suppose the target behavior is getting ready for school, but the child is not ready to put all of the steps together. The parent may want the child to start with the endpoint of success, namely walking into the school building alone. However, the child may get support for earlier steps in the sequence (walking to school, making breakfast, getting dressed, getting up on their own).

Internalization of Values

Though rewards and pleasing parents can help increase a child's motivation, the ultimate goal for parents is for their children to develop their own values that drive healthy behavior even when parents are not present. Ultimately, we hope that children will think for themselves, believe in the rules that they follow, and behave ethically. In helping parents look at the "long game," they may be able to see that helping their children build skills and self-esteem is more important than gaining immediate compliance.

Using questions, along with a reward system, can enhance the value and internalization: "Did you feel proud when you accomplished that?" "Did it feel good that you managed that situation without hitting" or "Is that something you want to do for yourself more than for getting a prize?"

Thoughts on Negative Consequences

Add punishments to the behavioral plan thoughtfully. An American Academy of Pediatrics policy statement (Sege & Siegel, 2018) notes that certain punishments, such as spanking, slapping, beating, and screaming, do more harm than good (see also Smith, 2012). When using appropriate punishments, such as active ignoring, removing reinforcement, and time-out, consider the dose of penalty. Make punishments specific, immediate, consistent, meaningful, and in balance. Make certain the parents know how to implement these interventions appropriately. For example, one parent reported that time-out "didn't work" because she had kept her child in his room for several days. When she was told that the general principle involved was a minute per year of age, she was surprised. She shifted her strategy and found that a shorter time-out was much more successful for her child.

Many parents scrutinize their children's interests for the purpose of removing favorite activities as a penalty. When parents want to make an impact, sometimes they impose a very big penalty. We have known several parents over the years who have, at the last minute, canceled their children's birthday parties as a punishment. One must wonder whether this penalty alters the child's behavior and, if so, in what ways. In the future, will the child remember the reason for the penalty or their feelings about their parents for imposing it? How does it affect the child's social standing with friends? Though parents are entitled to make these decisions, it is helpful to talk through the process with them. Punishments, when used, should be reserved for important behaviors. When implemented in the following ways, punishments may prove more beneficial.

- *Appropriate level of punishment.* Help the parents recognize that smaller penalties work better than larger ones, as they keep the focus on the child's behavior rather than on the penalty. The goal of the punishment should be to make the child recognize their behavior as incorrect and have the desire to fix it. If the endpoint is that they are enraged at their parents, the punishment has not met its goal. Considering ways to help the child regroup, such as waiting as the parent counts to 10 rather than going into a time-out, can be effective. Removing a misused toy for an hour, postponing screen time by an hour, or asking the child to complete an action to make amends (such as doing the dishes) can be effective.

- *Natural/logical consequences.* These exist in the world anyway. The key for parents may lie in not rescuing the child from the real-world implications of their behavior. An example is a child who dawdles on the way to school and is late: The child expects the parents to make an excuse to the school, but the parents do not and the lateness is noted. Or let's say that a child hits a friend and the friend responds by declining a playdate, the parent could have a discussion with the child rather than imploring the other parent to make their child forgive the incident.

- *Active ignoring.* Parents may benefit from instruction on active ignoring. They let the child know that they are not currently responding to their communications but do not further engage. An example might be, "I can't speak with you until you stop screaming," or the more positive "As soon as you use your indoor voice, we can talk." Active ignoring works best when the child understands what they have to do to regain the parent's attention. However, it is important to give the instruction only once and then not respond more. This can be hard for parents to carry out. If parents report that they have tried active ignoring and it did not work, you may need more information on implementation.

- *Apology of action, undoing the harm, and making a repair.* Teach parents about repair strategies. When children have done something wrong, sometimes they can make amends by demonstrating remorse or undoing the action. For example, if they break a toy, they can attempt to fix it or purchase a new item to replace what they broke. This strategy requires the postgame step of the child imagining the impact of their actions on others.

- *Don't lay down an ultimatum that you are not prepared to follow through on.* For parents, follow-through is important for both rewards and consequences. If the parent is going to take away the phone, for example, based on a behavior, they lose credibility if they do not follow through or if every punishment can be undone by earning back whatever was lost. This does not mean that a parent cannot be flexible. It does mean that every time an ultimatum is stated and not carried out, the child learns that those statements are meaningless. It is important *not* to follow through if the threat is dangerous, such as a threat to send the child to military school, or if the threat would lead to emotional harm. Before setting a punishment, the parents should imagine how they will succeed in delivering it. If the penalty is taking the child's phone, a very common one these days, how will the parent get the child to give it up? If it becomes a physical fight for the phone, this may not be the best plan for follow-through on that consequence. If the parent gets the phone but then gives it back because the child needs it to contact them after school, then the punishment becomes ineffective. Several parents who lack follow-through have reported that they do not act on the penalty because if they do "I will have nothing left to take away." Another reason that parents undo the punishment is based on the child's renewed positive behavior. Children soon understand that they can push their behavior to the edge, receive a penalty, and then undo it. This pattern also sustains negative behavior.

- *Rewinds.* If you want to help model flexibility, sometimes before a penalty is invoked or for more minor misbehaviors, the parent can ask the child to redo something they did not do well. A common example is a child who uses a whiny or babyish tone is asked by the parent to use a "big kid voice." When the child tries again in a better tone of voice, most often the parent delivers what they had requested. Though generally a good strategy, the goal should be to help the child to use more independent self-cues. "What voice should you use?" is one step closer, for example, to self-cueing. The parents should keep track of the pattern, because it may not decrease the use of whining. What it may do is simply add in a step: whine, cue, adjust voice.

This chapter provided an overview of the nuances in using behavioral techniques in parent guidance work. In the next part, we shift to discussing specific caregiver concerns and how to work with them.

WORKSHEET 12.1

Developing a Behavior Plan

Goal

- What is the behavioral goal?
- What behavior will get a reward in this plan?
- Is this an appropriate step toward the behavioral goal?
- Is this behavior doable for the child and one that the child has agreed to work on?

Reward

- What is the agreed-upon reward?
- Does the reward make sense for the behavior?
- Is it motivating for the child?
- Does the timing of the reward make sense for the developmental level of the child?
- Are the caregivers prepared to dispense the reward as agreed upon?

Setup

- How is the plan set up?
- Where will the plan be displayed?
- Does everyone understand it?
- How will successes be noted?

PART V

Specific Problems in the Caregiver

Imagine that a single mother contacts you regarding her 7-year-old son. She thinks he is anxious. You schedule an assessment session with the mother, who is very forthcoming in response to your questions. During the assessment you learn about the child, but you also learn that the mother is a high-powered lawyer, seemingly functioning very well. She tells you that, given her own anxiety disorder, her son's behavior upsets her tremendously. She does not know how to handle his anxiety and she winds up yelling. She is at her wits end, recognizing that her responses make things worse but unable to figure out what to do differently. Her mood is worsening. She knows she is not helping the situation. She asks how soon you will have your first appointment with her child. With whom do you schedule the appointment?

We have worked with many such parents, who seek our help in identifying problems to solve in their child. However, the best avenue for helping their child may be in changing the parent's response. Some caregivers are very open. Others are more insistent that the child make all of the changes. The chapters in this part of the book discuss strategies for the challenging work with caregivers that will improve child and family mental health.

CHAPTER 13

Helping the Caregiver Who Has Anxiety or Mood Regulation Issues

The Parent Has Anxiety That Impacts Parenting

There should be a diagnosis called "parental anxiety disorder." Parenting is not for the faint of heart, as children can make parents more anxious than just about anything else. If the caregiver has difficulty managing anxiety generated by having children, then parent guidance makes sense as an intervention. If the anxiety is more generalized, and impacting other areas of the caregiver's functioning, then individual therapy, either instead of or in addition to parent guidance is appropriate. What is the treatment strategy for our newly minted parental anxiety disorder? The following approach outlines the process for addressing parental anxiety.

STRATEGY: *Identify Sources of Anxiety and Reduce the Anxious Response.*

Identify the specific fears. Knowing what the parent's fears are is a logical first step in the process. There are a range of fears that typically accompany parenting. Be aware of the typical parental fears, including:

- Fear of being a "bad parent."
- Fear that the child will grow up to be a bad person (a disliked political figure, a criminal, a school shooter, the child's other parent), including the fear that the child may hurt someone.
- Fear that something will happen to the child in our dangerous world.
- Fear of making a choice that will lead to a terrible tragedy.
- Fear of missing opportunities by not knowing something or by not signing the child up for an activity. This includes the fear that their child will not get into a good college or attain a job that can pay enough to live on in our economy.

- Fear of repeating patterns from their family of origin.
- Fear that the child's current difficulties will never get better.
- Fear of major mental illness.
- Fear that taking medication will have dire consequences.

STRATEGY: *Engage in Cognitive Restructuring after Identifying the Fears*

The following three questions can help shift the fear into a more manageable range. These questions can be applied to all of the fears we have and begin a more action-oriented approach for the caregiver. There are no right or wrong answers to these questions. Rather, they help the caregiver gain distance by applying thoughts, rather than unprocessed fears, to alter feelings and generate realistic plans of action. The three questions are:

1. *How likely is it to happen (is it true)?* For example, suppose the parent has the fear that the child's difficulties will never get better. Help the parent evaluate whether this fear is likely to be true. If the child is in preschool and bites peers, the fear that this behavior will continue is very unlikely to be true, as this behavior often resolves with age. If the child is 17 years old, bites peers, and has an autism diagnosis, the behavior is more likely to persist and will need a targeted intervention.

2. *How serious would it be if it was a reality?* It is unlikely that the preschooler who bites will continue this behavior into adulthood. If they did, though, it would be fairly serious. For the teen with autism, this behavior may be very serious.

3. *What skills do I have for coping with this fear?* If the fear is rational and it would be serious if it were true, the next question is how the parent will manage both their feelings and the situation driving their fear. If the child is a biting teen, what would the parent do? What services would they put into place? How would they help the child? What could they do for themselves to better cope?

STRATEGY: *Reframe with the Parent*

Some parents judge themselves for having the fear in the first place, further complicating intervention attempts. Remind them that anxiety can be useful and protective, alerting people to dangers such as busy streets. A helpful reframe could be that their parental anxiety is an indicator that they love their child and that anxiety serves as an alarm to remind them to take action when necessary. However, when anxiety is too high, it also interferes with taking action and functioning well in daily life.

STRATEGY: *Stay in the Present*

Some caregiver fears focus on far-off outcomes, such as the fear that the child will never move out and support themself as an adult, although they are currently in elementary school. Reminding the caregiver to stay in the present moment or the near future helps to keep the solutions feasible. Ask the caregiver for evidence that supports their worry. If they are concerned that the child will be a serial killer or will be unsuccessful in life (according to their metrics), what makes them think so? Does the 5-year-old have a gun? Are they violent toward peers and adults? If the child's impulses lead to poor choices, can they be supervised more closely? What would be a next step to teach the child better interaction skills with peers? Ask the parent to focus on what they can do *now* to make the concerning outcome less likely.

STRATEGY: *Find Balance*

Help the parent find balance by thinking about areas other than having children, in which they have achieved life success. Some parents who worry about "doing parenting right" have been successful in many other arenas. This thought might lead them to conclude that, with effort, they can do a reasonable job raising a child. Help them recognize that everyone makes mistakes and that there is no clear path or one right way to be a parent to their child. Reducing comparisons with other parents, who often brag or post about their child's successes, can help as well. Remind parents that they have a life besides their child, and that their child too has their own life and choices.

STRATEGY: *Use Gradual Exposure*

Have the parent tolerate the fear about their child in small and reasonable doses. For example, if the parent is worried about the dangers in the world, allowing the child to have a sleepover with a friend or walk down the block while the parent watches can be a start.

STRATEGY: *Develop Supports*

Parents do not need to do everything. Are there people who have offered to help? What could they be helpful with? There are natural supports in people's lives that they may be able to access. There also may be more structured supports through school programs or social service agencies that would provide some relief or remove some burdens from a family. If a family can afford them, are there services that they can hire to remove some stress? Tutoring, housecleaning, babysitting, parent helpers, and even drivers can make a difference. Use Worksheet 13.1, "Who Else Can Help with My Daily Life?," to think through possible supports.

The Parent Has Mood Regulation Issues in the Context of Parenting

Often missing from the story the parents bring to you is how their own mood and anger outbursts contribute to interactions with their child. Parents may be surprised by the impact of their mood on the household, as young children mirror their parents' mood

(Aktar & Bogels, 2017). Do the caregivers understand what mood they are projecting and how that impacts others around them? When children are dysregulated and distressed, the upset can also have a contagious effect on the parent's mood. If you remind caregivers that remaining calm and resisting the contagion in the moment can shift the child's mood and also help themselves, they may be able to do it. Start with insight. When they understand what makes it difficult to effectively manage their mood, they can develop strategies that will help.

To put it another way, feedback is bidirectional. How many times, when walking down the street, did someone smile at you and it made you feel happy and return the smile? Similarly, if you meet someone who scowls, even if you do not know them, the expression can promote a shift in your own feelings and facial expressions. This is emotion contagion (Hatfield et al., 1993). Children are often keenly aware of parental mood. If caregivers experiment with their own projection of mood, they may be able to both generate more positive moments and also avoid intensifying negative situations.

In one example, Carlton, age 15, made dinner for the family. His mother had been very stressed about work and was projecting a lot of anger at home. Carlton thought making dinner would be helpful and expected that it would make his mother happy. Carlton did not, however, clean up well after he cooked the meal. There were dishes in the sink and food scraps on the counter. His mother, in a sarcastic tone, said, "Thanks for cleaning up." Carlton, who had been trying to please his mother, now became upset. He mirrored his mother's sarcastic style, sharply responding, "You're welcome for dinner. Remind me not to try and help again." The interaction went downhill from there. Had his mother been able to say, "Thanks for dinner. I really appreciate it," and, perhaps a bit later said, "Let's clean up together. The kitchen could use some work," she would have received a very different response.

We are closest to our family members emotionally, and it is easy to let our guard down with them. When situations feel out of control, caregivers can become upset, which perhaps manifests as yelling and disinhibition. Parents often feel guilty about these outbursts. At the same time, they may feel justified when the child has done something to precipitate an eruption. It is a difficult pattern to break. The parent's loss of control might shut down the child's negative behavior when they are frightened by the parent's reaction. The fact that the misbehavior stopped can either convince the parent that yelling works to get through to the child, or at least serves a reinforcing function of stopping the child, but not without some significant side effects to the child and the relationship.

Helping parents manage their own, often reasonable, emotions can create an immediate change in the pattern of conflict between parent and child. Though we might admit that little kids can sometimes be really difficult, we must convince parents to take the high road. Your task may be to remain empathic to the parent's situation even when they are behaving in unhelpful ways, acknowledging how hard it may be to be around an unreasonable child, to give up on one's own agenda, and to be treated in ways that would be considered abusive if the behavior occurred between two adults.

Help the Parent Identify Mood Dysregulation and Manage Feelings More Effectively

When you work with caregivers who become easily dysregulated, try this intervention approach:

- Increase the caregiver's self-awareness. Parents may not realize how often and seriously they lose their temper and yell at their children. Sometimes self-awareness is the only step needed to solve this issue.
- Educate the parent about the problems in this pattern, including the erroneous view that yelling and dysregulation help improve the child's behavior, when instead they may alienate and cause relationship problems.
- Help the parent better understand the precipitants or "buttons," for their reactions. If the parent simply becomes aware of what sets them off, they can then build coping skills and script preferable responses. They are more likely to carry out a different response if they have planned it when they are calm.
- Teach caregivers emotion regulation strategies. Work on a variety of skills, such as relaxation, taking a break, or stepping away from the situation. Additional specific emotion regulation skills, such as "stay STRONG" and "opposite action" are taught in DBT (Linehan, 2014). Developing these skills takes patience and persistence.
- When the problem is unhelpful thought patterns, identify the thoughts. Some of these thoughts may be reality based and others may be distortions, especially those about the child. If the parents believe, for example, that the child never listens to them, consider whether this is true and address cognitions that are faulty. The way people think affects how they feel, which is a basic tenet of CBT (Beck, 2020). If you can help the parent adjust their perspective and recognize the time-limited nature of their current struggles, often the behaviors and feelings will subsequently adjust.
- Teach the caregiver to use positive self-talk. Parents can narrate their own healthy responses to frustrating situations, such as telling themselves "I'm running late but it will be okay." Worksheet 13.2, "Positive Self-Talk for Parents," at the end of the chapter, can help with developing this skill.
- Celebrate when the parent demonstrates successful mood management. When they are unsuccessful, process what could have gone differently.
- Create a list of mantras for caregivers to use (Worksheet 13.3, "Useful Parent Mantras" provides examples). They can practice a few, keep some on a card that is easily accessible, or have one that is their go-to choice. "Let your mood lead the way" is an example of a useful mantra guiding the parent to exhibit a more positive affect.
- Provide psychoeducation about developmental aspects of battles with children. Children have little appreciation for historical context in relationships. For example, if they hit you 5 minutes ago, they may not understand why you are still

upset if they are now being nice. Teach the parents to use narration about these interactional consequences, while allowing the situation to return to normal. "I'll calm down in a minute, but I am still thinking about how you hit" or "It is great that you calmed your body down now. How can you keep from hitting again?" These scripts that you share with parents can be very useful, since it can be challenging to come up with helpful language in the heat of the moment.

- Remind parents about the value in the postgame. Sometimes parents are so distressed about the child's behavior that they have trouble returning to baseline or "normal," and instead keep the fight going with their own dysregulated mood and behavior. Once parents have returned to their baseline mood, they can discuss the situation with the child. The child is more likely to acknowledge their own contribution to a difficult situation if they are discussing it after the fact with a calm parent.
- Parents may regret what they say in the midst of battles with their children, though sometimes they do not! Children hold on to what is said in anger ("I wish I never had kids."), even when parents have forgotten. When parents have problems with impulse control, self-awareness, and empathy, it can help the therapist to remember that the parents are probably trying their best but are struggling as well. Take up the challenge of remaining empathic to the parent, providing them with perspective about what they have said and, at the same time, nonjudgmentally help determine what to do or say instead.
- Sometimes parents are frustrated and have lost hope about their child's behavior or their relationship with their child. Inspire caregivers to retain a realistic hope for change. Parents benefit when they see that you are "with them" in solving the problems with their children. Explicitly let them know that you remain hopeful for them, while they struggle to believe that things can change.
- Parental mood dysregulation can exist in the context of very busy lives. A newspaper survey finds that parents get about 32 minutes of free time a day (Schmall, 2018). Remind them that you know that they matter too. When a negative event occurs with their child, you can help them understand that the process of change is a jagged, not linear, path.

Worksheets 13.2, "Positive Self-Talk for Parents"; 13.3, "Useful Parent Mantras"; 13.4, "I Am Angry/Dysregulated (and It's Not Helping)"; and 13.5, "Self-Care for Parents" can be used to help improve affect management in parents.

WORKSHEET 13.1

Who Else Can Help with My Daily Life?

Person/Role*	What Can They Help With?**

*Could be a co-parent, grandparent, family friend, coach, babysitter, church friend, among others. Cast a wide net when thinking about this choice.

**Could involve giving you a break, helping with homework, being the person your child can open up to, or taking you out for a fun moment when you need to get away. There are many different things someone else can help with.

WORKSHEET 13.2

Positive Self-Talk for Parents

Example:
I've got this.

Example:
My children love me.

WORKSHEET 13.3

Useful Parent Mantras

- "Children do well if they can" (Greene, 1998).
- Parents do well if they can.
- It's a skills deficit.
- Let your mood lead the way.
- You get what you model.
- You get what you give.
- Don't take the bait.
- Practice patience.
- Practice listening.
- Teach skills, not obedience.
- Model flexibility.
- It's a stage.
- Beam warmth.
- "Astonish [ourselves] with love." (Kornfield, n.d.)
- My child is so beautiful when they are asleep [and go look at them while they are sleeping].
- Forget the mistake, remember the lesson.
- Be the change you want to see (often attributed to Mahatma Gandhi).
- Be your own sunshine.
- Keep it simple.
- Awareness precedes change.
- Every journey starts with a single step.
- Dream big and don't be afraid to fail.

WORKSHEET 13.4

I Am Angry/Dysregulated (and It's Not Helping)

How do I know?	What can I do immediately so I don't make the situation worse?
What can I do in the medium term (later that day)?	**What can I do in the long term?**

WORKSHEET 13.5

Self-Care for Parents

What can I do **in the moment** to help me feel good about how I managed myself in the situation?

What can I do **in the moment** to keep the situation from getting worse?

What can I do **in the moment** to pause and feel better?

____

____

____

____

____

What can I do **shortly after** to feel calmer?

What can I do **shortly after** to enjoy myself?

What can I do **shortly after** to improve my mood?

____

____

____

____

____

What can I do in the **long term** to manage myself and my emotions well?

What can I do in the **long term** to take care of myself physically and emotionally?

What can I do in the **long term** to enjoy myself, my children, and my life?

____

____

____

____

____

CHAPTER 14

Helping the Caregiver When There Is a Relationship Problem with the Child

The Reciprocal Nature of the Caregiving Relationship

Interactions between the caregiver and child change both members of the dyad. Who the child is will impact the nature of the parenting, as it is an inherently reciprocal relationship, as described by Sameroff's (2009) transactional model. A parent may intend to have many rules, but find that their child is cautious and needs little imposed structure. Another caregiver may be more laid-back, but then have a child who benefits from more structure. These examples describe situations in which a parent makes a decision to adjust their style to meet the needs of their child. Perhaps more often, the transactions between the parent and child modify the style of the parent without that caregiver making a conscious decision.

Parent–Child Relationship Problem

The most important relationship here, the relationship that needs to develop and remain strong, is the one between the caregiver and the child (Scheeringa & Zeanah, 2001; Lieberman & Van Horn, 2011). Some problems in the relationship manifest as mismatches, lack of trust for one another, consistent unpleasant interactions, lack of collaboration, lack of joy in general, and not finding ways to spend pleasurable time together. These areas are where the real work lies. Regardless of other identified emotional and behavioral goals, improvement in all goal areas is more likely when there is a strong foundational caregiving relationship. When there is a parent–child relationship problem, the caregiver needs help in evolving from being part of the problem to becoming a catalyst for positive change. The relationship will need repair or improvement before other interventions will be effective.

Step back and think about the work we are doing to develop the relationship between the parent and child. Interventions that are not directly focused on the relationship may still lead to improvement in that area. We may be using behavioral interventions but when those behavioral interventions improve the situation, the parent and child enjoy spending more time together. This has a beneficial synergistic effect. Caregivers will have more positive moments with their child and will feel more confident in setting limits and addressing behavioral concerns. Children will enjoy their parents more and, because of the enhanced relationship, will be more interested in pleasing their parents.

STRATEGY: *Consider the Match between the Child's Needs and the Parent's Style*

A child may have a difficult temperament (Gartstein et al., 2012). Or the child may have attentional concerns or another concern that makes them more challenging to raise than another child. Now imagine that the child's parents struggle with their own executive functioning or other parenting skills. This constitutes a mismatch between the child's needs and the parents' abilities. Another child may have a calm demeanor and an easy temperament. That child will not likely have significant troubles, regardless of the parents' skill level in managing challenging behavior. The child with the difficult temperament may do better behaviorally if they have a parent with better skills.

When talking about the work with parents, referencing this idea of the match between the child's needs and the caregiver's parenting style is helpful because there is no blame involved. Help the parents understand what you mean using examples, for example, a parent may be artistic but have a child who has no interest in art. This parent would benefit from finding and supporting their child's strengths, rather than by pushing the child to be more like them. Increase the caregiver's motivation to change by recognizing the impact of the mismatch on the child. Progress can occur when the parent recognizes where the mismatch is and makes an active plan to diminish its impact.

Expectations and Attributions

"My daughter walked out of class. She just loves causing trouble." In sessions with caregivers you may find yourself thinking, "That explanation of their child's behavior does not really make sense." Some parents have explanations for their child's behavior that are unrealistic, upset the parent, and set them up for negative interactions because they are assuming the worst, rather than the best, intentions from their child.

Unrealistic Expectations

Sometimes parents wish that their children would behave differently even when the child's behavior is developmentally typical. That said, many typical behaviors can be annoying and are especially noticeable during the preschool and teen years, when normative behavior can be very challenging, such as the risk taking that teens sometimes engage in. Unrealistic expectations can also occur when the parent wishes for their child to excel in ways that are not possible for the child nor of interest to them.

STRATEGY: *Identify the Unrealistic Expectations and Bring Them into More Realistic Ranges*

When you assess that the parent has unrealistic expectations for the child, either because of a lack of understanding of typical development or because of their own dreams for the child, follow these approaches:

- Identify the expectation and its likelihood of being met. If the caregiver wishes for their child to be toilet trained at 5 months of age, that expectation is not realistic. Some expectations are unrealistic for any child of a given age. You can also assess whether the expectation is reasonable for this particular child. If a child does not yet put on their own pants, it is unlikely that they will be able to fully dress themselves tomorrow, even when other same age children already do so.

- Provide the caregiver with education about child development and how it progresses. Discuss developmental patterns. If you talk about how a child may stand before they walk, the caregiver may then understand that their child has to develop words for their feelings before they can express them, which is a completely different behavior but one that analogously develops in steps.

- Get the backstory about the unrealistic expectation. If the parent expects the child to have perfect table manners at age 5, why is this important? Does the parent wish to be able to go out to fancier restaurants where good table manners would be required? Was the parent themself raised with very strict expectations around table manners? If the wish is for the child to be the quarterback, did the parent play football? How did their love for football come about?

- Find out about the child's expectations. Does the child share the caregiver's expectation and join in the mission to make it happen? Or does the child push back? Does it hurt the child's self-esteem to be encouraged and expected to do something out of their reach?

- Consider asking these three questions when it is helpful.
  1. *Is the expectation reasonable?* Will the child be toilet trained at 5 months? Will they take some risks as a teenager? Can they be the high school quarterback? The answer will depend on the child, their interests, and their abilities.
  2. *How serious would it be if the child does not meet the expectation?* Here again the caregiver has to answer this question for themselves. You can help them process their response and address both their helpful and unhelpful cognitions.
  3. *What coping skills does the caregiver have?* What can they do if the child does not yet, or will not ever, meet the goal? If the goal is for their child to have good table manners because the parent would like to go to fancy restaurants, can

the caregiver's need be met another way, such as by hiring a babysitter so the parent can have an evening on their own?

- If the expectation is about a skill the child does not yet have, help the caregiver find incremental ways to teach the skill. Identify smaller steps to take along the way and how the parent can help the child move through those steps successfully.

Parental Attributions about Their Children

Parents' attributions may contribute to the overall dynamic, maintaining a child's challenging behavior. Attributions, in this case, have to do with what someone thinks is the cause of a behavior or characteristic. Behavior does not occur in isolation. It usually follows feelings and attributions. In their landmark study of resiliency, Werner and Smith (1992) report that the most predictive variable for a child's positive outcome was the mother's rating, when the child was 2 years old, of "lovability." This rating may say more regarding the mother's attributions about the child than about the child's actual traits.

Explore, with caregivers, whether they are making automatic attributions about their child's behavior that may upset them and lead to less helpful responses. Help parents recognize that how they think and feel about and view their child's behavior has an impact on the child. Determine whether a caregiver's attribution about their child's behavior is realistic, developmentally appropriate, and helpful. Some parents will say that their toddler is "manipulative" or is "trying to upset" them. We have heard parents imply that their infant is deliberately making them angry. Even older children are unlikely to be trying to make their parents angry. Consider this example:

PARENT: Kevin has left his book at school twice this week. He knows what a pain it is for me to have to drive him back there and get it when I am trying to make dinner. He just doesn't care about me. It really pisses me off. I do so much for him, and he doesn't even think about me.

THERAPIST: So some of what is bugging you about this is that you think he doesn't care about you?

PARENT: Well . . . he cares about me, but it sure feels like he doesn't when he does things like this.

THERAPIST: One explanation of this behavior is that he just doesn't care. I wonder if, given his age, and his diagnosis of ADHD, it is really hard for him to remember to go over to the bin where they keep the reading books and get his book at the end of the day.

PARENT: Maybe.

THERAPIST: Maybe we need to help figure out a system to make it more likely that the book will wind up in his backpack. Perhaps his teacher can help. Maybe his inattention is the culprit rather than his not caring about you.

PARENT: That's true. Some other system would probably work better because this one is not working for either of us!

The parent is not likely aware that they are making assumptions when they verbalize attributions about their child's behavior, nor do they realize how their attributions impact their feelings and interactions. Adjust attributions by bringing them to awareness, examining the likelihood that they are accurate or the only possibility, and offering alternative explanations. Help parents discern what the attribution is doing. Is it helpful in the situation or inflaming it?

STRATEGY: *Explain Attributions and Work to Change Them*

Once parents are aware of their attributions, help them to develop more understanding ones as possibilities and see if this shift changes the caregivers' affect and behavior toward their child. The parent is not likely aware that they are making assumptions when they verbalize attributions about their child's behavior, nor do they realize how their attributions impact their feelings and interactions. Provide education about attributions.

Help caregivers brainstorm other potential attributions about their child's behavior. Offer examples of situations in which a person could make different attributions about the reasons for a behavior and then what the ensuing feelings and interactions would be like. You might start with examples applicable to the parent. Ask them to imagine that they are walking down the hall at work and they pass a friend. The friend does not say hello. Have the parent talk about what they assume the reason is, talk through or offer alternative explanations, and identify how each explanation would lead the caregiver to feel and behave.

Do the same exercise with the child's behavior. Have the parent identify a scenario and walk through different possible attributions. Perhaps the child takes 30 minutes to do a 5-minute chore. The parent gets angry, thinking that the child is thoughtless and does not care what the rest of the family needs to do. Brainstorm other possibilities: Attentional difficulties, poor fine motor skills, and underdeveloped executive functions would all explain the behavior without suggesting that the child is thoughtless about the rest of the family. How many explanations can they derive for what their child is doing? Worksheet 14.1, "Attributions," offers a framework to help caregivers think through the possibilities.

Teaching Relationship Skills, Including Validation and Attunement

There are many strategies that strengthen the parent–child relationship in addition to managing attributions. Multiple therapeutic approaches focus on validation, at least as one important tool. For example, we see this in collaborative and proactive solutions (CPS; Greene, 1998) and in parent–child interaction therapy (PCIT; McNeil & Hembree-Kigin, 2010). Validation means communicating that the caregiver hears and accepts what their child is feeling. Another tool, attunement, involves the parent understanding what the child is communicating, even when the child is not saying in words what they are feeling, and then responding to the needs of the child. One mother overheard her preadoptive daughter talking to friends and being mean. It was the end of the school year, and the teen would not be returning to this school in the fall. This intuitive parent thought to herself, "She's 'breaking up' with them so that the separation is easier for her." This was a child with significant loss and separation in her history. With that understanding, the mother was able to resist talking about it on the ride home, giving the teen some space. At a later time, she brought up with the girl that it was probably really hard for her to leave the school. She did not say, "You were really mean to your friends. What's up with that?" Instead, she understood what was motivating the behavior and approached it in an empathic way, leading to a productive conversation.

For parent–child relationship concerns, try these interventions:

- Identify ways the relationship problem manifests itself. Do problems occur all of the time? Is there a focus for the difficulties?
- Find times when the relationship works better. Help the caregiver move beyond all-or-nothing thinking. There have probably been some times in the child's life when, at least momentarily, the relationship went better. What did those times have in common? Find the links and opportunities for caregivers to recreate times when the relationship worked more smoothly.
- Help the caregiver find ways to relate to the child at the child's level. Improve the relationship through child-led play and teen-led interaction, which are important and sometimes sufficient to shift a negative dynamic. These interventions are often used to improve relationships in general and can be a good boost to any intervention, as described in depth in Part II, Chapter 5. In fact, a number of evidence-based models, such as PCIT, use this technique.
- Help the parent identify enjoyable activities that they can do with their child. Perhaps there are shows or movies that they both would like. Would the child like to be read to by the parent? Are there places they both like to go? Come up with a list and help them plan when to engage in some of these pursuits.
- Help the caregiver find ways to be more positive. Relationship problems are rare for people who are complimentary about themselves and others, have bright affect, and find positive things in the world. It would be especially beneficial if the caregiver was, at times, positive with their child.
- Help the caregiver reframe their narrative. Describe the problem as separate from the child, for example, a child who is angry as opposed to an angry child.
- There are interventions that are geared toward improving attachment, such as the Circle of Security, which was developed by Powell et al. (2016). This intervention focuses on building a secure attachment with the parent. Through an assessment process of figuring out the dyadic pattern, the therapist can create an individualized approach to fostering empathy between the parent and child. Parents are taught to read child cues and develop appropriate responses. In parent guidance, the caregiver can learn concepts from attachment theory, such as the importance of reading cues, developing a secure base from which a child can explore, and providing comfort to a distressed child.

Interventions Designed to Build Validation Skills

Validation involves nonjudgmentally communicating that the caregiver understands what the child is saying. It can deescalate situations because the child feels heard and therefore does not have to work harder to communicate. To improve parental validation skills, try the following interventions:

- Teach the parent the importance of validation. Ask them to come up with examples of when they did not feel validated, such as with their own parents, a romantic partner, or in a conversation with a professional such as a physician. Have them reflect on how not being validated made them feel and what they wanted to do in response.
- Teach the parent how to validate their child's feelings. If the caregiver has a sense of what their child is feeling, they can reflect it back and let their child know that they understand that the child is feeling that way. Role play examples of the child's statements and validating responses with parents who struggle to find the words.
- Give the caregiver examples and scripts that they can adapt to their circumstances.
- Remind the caregiver that they may need to validate more than they feel is necessary in order for the child to feel heard, especially before they move into problem solving.

Worksheet 14.2, "Understanding Validation," can help caregivers learn about this skill.

Improving Attunement Skills

Attunement is about "reading" the child's behaviors, even when they are not stating their feelings explicitly. For example, if the child comes home from school, goes into their room, and slams the door, the attuned parent might think "something happened at school or on the bus." Knowing their child well, they would then choose to either approach the child and ask them if they want to talk or give them some time by themselves if that is what works well for that particular child. A parent who is not attuned might think that the child's behavior is really rude, yell at the child for slamming the door, and tell them to come out of their room.

Blaustein and Kinniburgh (2010) discuss attunement as being able to "accurately read each other's cues and respond appropriately" (p. 65). These cues may be revealed in the form of behaviors, communication, or needs. Many children do not communicate what is going on for them in a well-reasoned and clear way. Instead, they may communicate it with difficult behaviors or challenging interactions. The caregivers' capacity to read what is prompting such behaviors allows for a more helpful and proactive response. To build attunement skills, we suggest the following approaches:

- The parent can work specifically on reading their child's cues. During your sessions ask the parent for examples of the child's behavior and talk them through how to do this. Help the caregiver be a detective looking for an understanding of why their child does what they do. With perspective taking, they can respond in more helpful ways.
- Brainstorm, with the caregiver, developmental and affective factors that could contribute to the child's behavior. For example, if a child has experienced trauma, they may startle at seemingly innocuous stimuli, such as a door slamming. Talking through triggers may help the caregiver more accurately identify the reasons for a child's behavior.
- Help the caregiver identify regularly occurring vulnerability factors for their child, such as hunger, inadequate sleep, situational anxiety, and emotionally charged events. Once they are identified, coach caregivers to take these factors into account when considering the reasons for their child's behavior.
- Use Worksheet 14.3, "Reading My Child's Behavior," helps develop this skill.

In summary, when working on developing attunement skills, caregivers can try to ask themselves the following questions when interpreting their child's behavior:

"What is my child doing?"
"What might be prompting that behavior?"
"How can I respond given what might be prompting the behavior?"

When the Parent Has Significant Negative Feelings about Their Child

The last parent–child relationship problem we cover in this chapter is the fact that parents do not always like their children. Negative feelings about a child can be uncomfortable to observe, especially for a therapist. The first step here may be acceptance that these feelings can occur. The next step is to be committed to changing this situation.

STRATEGY: *Accept That Parents Can Have These Feelings and That They Can Change over Time*

Clinicians need to be both supportive and bold in conversations about difficult thoughts and feelings caregivers have. It can be a relief to parents when they know that they are not alone in feeling that they do not enjoy, love, or want their child.

When caregivers express a dislike for their child, broach this topic carefully and with empathy. It demonstrates that you are willing to talk about topics that feel taboo. It also does lead to potential changes in goals. For example, the focus can quickly pivot to developing the relationship and the desire to be with this other person. Or the focus can become pragmatically thinking about what the next steps will be. Overall, though, communication needs to be both compassionate and fearless. In order to address the more serious negative feelings that a parent has for their child, we offer the following suggestions:

- Approach these conversations rather than shying away from them. Let parents know it is important to figure out how to tackle these feelings and do so in a nonjudgmental way. Recognize that shame is a significant part of these dialogues.

- Plan to spend ongoing sessions with the caregiver dealing with this concern. It is not a quickly and easily resolved topic.

- Recognize the feeling. Sometimes allowing parents to confess that they feel this way is, perhaps, counterintuitively, a great relief to them and provides a forum to begin addressing it. When parents hear that they are not alone in feeling unhappy with their child, they can often then gain the energy to take an active approach to modifying their feelings. It can also be helpful when you explain that although they feel this way now, they may not feel this way forever.

  Do not move away from this feeling too quickly; it can be invalidating to swiftly shift to a new topic. The bravery involves hearing the sentiment, in full, including potential ramifications. For some families the experience of having children was not what they expected; the child had significant behavioral and emotional challenges, or parenting just was not as rewarding as anticipated. We have seen families fall apart or formally disrupt, as in foster and adoptive situations. In those situations, once you have tried, for example, intensive therapies and respite services, you will need to help the caregiver through this process in a way that is as gentle as possible.

- Identify times with the parent when they find something endearing or engaging about the child. If the feeling is entrenched, it may help them to see the child through someone else's eyes, if that does not make the parent feel guilt or shame.

- Help the parent identify appropriate ways to behave regardless of their feelings. Caregivers may wish to avoid time with the child and, indeed, time away that is fulfilling to them may be an important component for doing better. That said, the parent may have to "fake it" until their feelings for the child become more positive.

- Script ways to talk and behave. Given that the parent's impulses and feelings are not positive toward the child, they may need to think in advance about healthier ways to react, interact, and speak with them. The parent may appreciate a script with ways to say something neutral or positive to use when their feelings about their child are mostly negative.

- The parent may dislike the child because they believe that the child does not like them, particularly if the child behaves in angry or sarcastic ways. Script responses for the parent that will, at least, not make the situation worse and, over time, may improve the relationship. One possibility is "I know we don't always get along perfectly, but I am always on your side."

- The parent may express resentment at being the one to have to make this change, especially when their child is behaving in seemingly unreasonable ways. Help them understand that, while that is a natural thought, they are more likely to bring about change if they initiate the effort.

Many problems seem to be solved when there are improvements in the relationship between the caregiver and the child. Think of these tools for understanding and intervening as first-line approaches when the relationship is a primary concern. The next chapter more explicitly addresses the caregiver who makes the problem worse.

WORKSHEET 14.1

Attributions

Example of what my child did	I automatically thought it was because . . .	A more helpful or realistic thought would be . . .
My toddler screamed when I wouldn't give her ice cream.	She is manipulative.	She is young and has not learned about healthy eating yet. She's just trying to get her wants met.

WORKSHEET 14.2

Understanding Validation

Why do it?

(Example: Improves relationship)

How can I communicate validation/be validating?

(Example: "That stinks that your friend said that.")

What will I do if it doesn't go well?

(Example: "Maybe he just needs some space right now.")

WORKSHEET 14.3

Reading My Child's Behavior

What is my child doing?

What might be behind this behavior?

How can I respond given what might be behind this behavior?

CHAPTER 15

Helping the Caregiver Who Makes the Problem Worse

Many parental actions inflame emotional and behavioral problems in children. These caregivers actively, though unintentionally, worsen their child's behavior. They may lack the skills to be more effective, or they may put in effort but be ineffectual, not knowing what will be helpful or not being able to follow through. Skill building is the key intervention strategy for these parents.

The Caregiver Who Lacks Skills

Entrenched Patterns of Interaction to Identify and Change

We all have repeated patterns of behavior that are entrenched or habitual and challenging to change. Habits, in this context, may include repeating the same unhelpful phrases ("What's wrong with you?") or becoming very angry at small infractions. These types of habits actively make it harder for the child to achieve their emotional or behavioral goals, often despite the parents desperately wanting the child to change.

One common pattern is making threats to get children to behave: "There's no TV if . . ." or "I'll take your phone away if. . . ." When helping these families, pay attention to both what they are not doing and also to what they are already doing. One caregiver could only stop his own yelling when his children cried and when he saw that they were remorseful and sad. Once he gained insight, he was able to shift the pattern to reduce his yelling. There is an oft-repeated loop that starts with difficult child behavior and moves to parent yelling and finally to child crying and sometimes to parent apology, only to restart without resolution or change.

STRATEGY: *Identify and Change Parental Habits*

Get detailed examples from caregivers of how the difficult interactions go. Determine whether there are repeated patterns of interacting that are contributing to the child's difficulties. When you believe that the parent has developed an ineffective or harmful habit, you can use the systematic strategy we discuss in the following sections.

Identify the Problematic Habit

By asking thorough questions about the regularly occurring family interactions you discover patterns that the caregivers are not aware of. When the caregiver describes the same sequence happening repeatedly, follow this clue. Remember that habits are not only ways of behaving, but also involve saying the same phrases, thinking similar thoughts, and having the same feelings repeatedly. Targeted questions about what the caregiver does, what they think and how they feel, will aid in identifying patterns. For example, a parent may describe the daily homework routine: The child comes home from school, throws their backpack on the floor in the living room, and runs to their room to play a computer game. The caregiver sees the backpack on the floor and is immediately angry.

CAREGIVER: Haven't I told you a million times to empty your lunch box? What do you have for homework?

CHILD: I did it all at school.

CAREGIVER: (*Checks the online communication system and finds that the child has not completed homework for many days.*)

CAREGIVER: What about math?

CHILD: I told you I already did it.

CAREGIVER: (*Looks in the backpack and finds many unfinished assignments.*) Turn off that game right now and start your homework.

CHILD: You're the worst parent ever! (*Screams and cries, throwing items around the room.*)

CAREGIVER: That's it! No games for the rest of the week!

If this sort of interaction happens regularly, the parent may have developed the following habits: gearing up for an argument in the afternoon, becoming angry at the child after school, asking the child questions about homework that elicit lies, checking on the child's truthfulness, yelling, and then delivering a consequence that is unlikely to be enforced or to effectively alter the child's homework behavior or mood. Does this same sort of dialogue and predictable behavior occur in the families that you see? Once you identify these patterns of behavior, you can also identify the habits of each family member. When the parent is more self-aware, you help them to shift into more effective, skill-building strategies for themselves and their child.

Build Self-Awareness about the Habit

It is amazing how often people are unaware of their own typical ways of responding. Once you start to understand the family's habitual ways of interacting, nonjudgmentally share your observations about these exchanges. When the caregiver understands that they have an unhelpful habit, they can consider whether they would like to change.

Increase the Parent's Interest in Change

People have trouble altering habits even when they are not working. Asking the simple question "Is that working for you?" or "Is that how you'd like it to be?" can move people toward change. Help them understand how this pattern is playing out and not leading to their desired outcomes. Ask how hard it would be to do something differently. What are the barriers? Motivational interviewing techniques (Frey & Hall, 2021) and the transtheoretical model (Prochaska & DiClemente, 1983) utilize the concept of stages of change, which is helpful when the caregiver feels stuck. For example, when someone is not ready to quit smoking, giving them techniques to quit will not bring about change. Similarly, if a parent is not ready to change their caregiving habits, then throwing ideas at them to try will also not bring about change. Assess their readiness to do things differently, determine what might provide motivation, and move them along a change trajectory. Sometimes parents are enthusiastic about trying something new, but the concept of making a change feels threatening or daunting.

Some parents feel that if the child is lying or misbehaving, getting angry and applying consequences are the only reasonable responses. They may be entrenched in this way of responding, not only because it is a habit, but also because they, and/or those around them, feel that responding this way is correct. Focus on what is effective, not on what is correct or ideal. For example, it is likely that what they want is for the child to tell the truth. Direct the parents' attention to that goal and then work toward responses that will help them achieve that goal. Let them know that, while being truthful is certainly an important value to instill in children, you can start with improving the child's behavior and then over time attend to telling the truth. Improve interactions, and truthfulness is more likely to follow.

Identify the Lagging Skill

An ineffective habit may be perpetuated by a lack of other ideas or abilities. Some of the reasons why people parent the way they do is because they lack a more expansive repertoire.

Identify Replacement Behaviors

Once the parent is aware of their behavior, is interested in changing it, and has the skill to monitor and adjust their behavior, you can help them identify a new replacement behavior or habit. There are many other possible ways that the after-school interaction between parent and child could play out in the previous example. For example, the caregiver could do one of the following:

- Add in, at the outset, a more positive way to start the interaction, such as greeting the child, asking the child how their day went, or offering a snack.
- Create a better pattern regarding the lunch box and backpack as soon as the child walks in the door by using a visual checklist or simple and calm verbal reminders.
- Slow down and be thoughtful about the timing of the sensitive question. Wait before asking the child to do homework, recognizing that the child may need a break before being confronted about their behavior.
- Stop the ineffective behavior of using threats and yelling. If the caregiver is not yet able to do something else, work with them on pausing before responding.
- Implement concrete strategies. Help the parent wonder why the child is behaving in a certain way and consider new ways to tackle the homework problem.

Address the Caregiver's Feelings That Get in the Way of Effective Responses

Sometimes parents behave poorly because they have their own intense feelings. Wonder with the parent about why they feel as they do. Parents may need to hear from the provider that parenting is difficult and often depriving. If they resent their children, validate the feelings and think about the cognitions that drive these feelings. If the parent's response to feelings is a "yelling habit," work with them to see the impact of this automatic response on themselves, their child, and their family. More significant affect management is addressed in the next section.

If the parent's response is to withdraw, help them recognize and understand the impact of that dynamic and offer alternative responses, including self-talk, slowing down, and reframing cognitions. Possible helpful cognitions include "She doesn't know how to put her backpack away yet"; "I was older when I started remembering to do these things"; or "I'll give him a second to get settled and then I can remind him." If the parent's intense feelings relate to stressors in their life that do not have to do directly with the child, help them recognize that these feelings are affecting their parenting.

The Parent Has Poor Boundaries

Another entrenched issue is a lack of boundaries on the caregiver's part. Examples include parents sharing embarrassing details about their children's lives with other people or becoming friends with their teenagers' friends. Boundary issues arise when parents are not able to differentiate their children's roles in the family from their own. The strategy is to provide education about boundaries and how they evolve as the child grows.

- If the parents were raised without appropriate boundaries, it may be harder for them to understand the concept. Provide examples and explanations of healthy boundaries, such as a teen wanting to shut their door and why they might do so.
- Offer alternative behaviors so that the caregiver has another option at the ready

when they otherwise would have committed a boundary violation. Talk about resisting the urge to barge into their child's room or read their child's diary. Discuss both the temptation and the reasons why, unless there is a strong provocation to engage in these behaviors, these violations should be resisted.

- Boundaries adjust as children grow. Prepare caregivers for changing their expectations as their children age. How will the parent cope with allowing their child increasing responsibility and freedom? How will they balance privacy and safety concerns with their teenagers?

The Caregiver Had Poor Parental Role Models

For parents who experienced problematic caregiving when they were young, they may want to do a better job than their own parents did but not know how.

STRATEGY: *Educate Caregivers about the Role of Upbringing and Modeling on How People Parent and about How to Change*

As caregivers consider how they were parented, they will start to realize how their own internal working models developed and to think about what they would like to keep and change as parents. Reflecting on their own upbringing removes shame while giving parents an understanding of why they do what they do. Many caregivers are eager to connect the dots from their upbringing, attachment to caregivers, and internal working models of parenting to their hope of becoming the parents they wish to be. When their own personal experience has included mostly negative models, they can look to other caregivers, real and fictional, as representations of what they would like to strive for. Use Worksheets 15.1, "Parent Values," and 15.2, "Model of an Ideal Parent," to help caregivers identify their parenting values and what they consider to be positive parenting.

Use parents' responses on these worksheets to identify what they want to do differently, the values that they want to embody as a parent, and the barriers to being the caregiver they ideally want to be. What would changes look like? How would they know if they are parenting differently? What do they need to put into place to make that happen? Get concrete with them in terms of strategies and then help them monitor changes they make.

The Parent Is Ineffective in Helping Their Child Improve

Like children, parents would do well if they could. They would use a broader range of behaviors if they were available to them. What skills do we think parents need to learn to do well in their parenting role? Caregivers are doing the best they can, but need you to help them parent differently.

When a child is struggling, their caregiver may need more than the basic skills required of a parent. Self-awareness, empathy and perspective taking, frustration management, and the ability to understand what their child's behavior is communicating can make an enormous difference in changing the family system. Working with caregivers on the following skills will help them become more effective in helping their child improve.

Self-Awareness

Many people, caregivers included, lack awareness of their own contributions to difficult situations. Some caregivers are aware only of the intention of their behaviors, rather than the impact of them. These same caregivers might be hypervigilant to every (negative) detail of their child's behavior and focus exclusively on the child's contributions to the difficult interaction. Low self-awareness perpetuates negative patterns of behavior by contributing to distortions and curtailing the opportunity to recognize the value in parental change. By analyzing how situations unfold as the caregiver describes them, you can, in a supportive manner, call attention to the ways in which their behavior led to some of the outcomes and help develop self-awareness.

Inhibiting Behaviors That Worsen the Situation

There are many typical parent no-nos that cannot be taken back, such as physical aggression, including slaps, which model poor coping and can cross the line to abuse. There are also verbal no-nos such as threats to send the child away ("You're going to jail/the hospital/boarding school/military school"), comments about how the child negatively impacted the parent's life ("Why did I ever have kids," "You're ruining my life," or "You're just like [disliked relative, such as other parent]"). When you ask parents, they will often offer that they have said one of these things.

These lapses can be a source of shame for the parent. Be careful not to have a judgmental tone when discussing them, as parents often struggle with finding appropriate alternatives that they can use. Brainstorming and role playing with the parents are effective ways to teach healthier responses. Caregivers often enjoy practicing conversations, role playing as their child, to entrap the therapist in the same impossible situations that they struggle with. Generate, with them in session, phrases to say, such as "I am REALLY angry right now" and "I need to take some space." Let parents know that they can express difficult sentiments in a frustrated and angry tone of voice, but without yelling in an out-of-control manner. You can also augment your role play by analyzing: "Why would he say that?"; "Why do you think she does that?"; "Am I responding as you would?"

Frustration Tolerance

Building frustration tolerance is a skill most caregivers could benefit from. Find out how parents manage frustration and help them to create strategies to use when they are most upset. Help them learn to recognize the signs that they are becoming frustrated. Self-talk around managing frustration can help them to develop this skill. Create a set of steps that the caregiver can employ when feeling frustrated, which may be similar to the ones described in the next section on lowering the thermostat.

Lowering the Thermostat

Help parents to walk away from a conflict when continuing is not productive and they choose to intervene at a later point. Identify a place for caregivers to go to "reset" when they are upset. Work with them to come up with very concrete strategies that they can use to take space or calm themselves. They might involve listening to music (have a specific song in mind and have it readily available), using a mindfulness exercise that they have practiced and find helpful, using activities from a coping box that they have created, doing breathing exercises, blowing bubbles, or using other specific skills designed to shift emotions. Some people benefit from more active ways to alter how they are feeling: Would this parent benefit from listening to loud music and dancing? Shooting some hoops? Going for a run? Doing push-ups?

Perspective Taking for the Child's Situation

In addition to expanding the caregivers' understanding of their own behavior, zooming in on the child's perspective can build empathy, shifting the tone of parent–child interactions. One parent complained about what a difficult week he had with his child. While recounting his experience, he noted that the child said she did not feel well; every day she said she did not want to go to school, stalling and making the morning difficult. The parent also noted that his daughter had a fever one day and could not go to school. This is a child who often said she did not feel well, so the father dismissed her concerns. He then continued to complain about the difficulty of the week. The therapist asked if he thought the daughter's behavior related to being sick, based on the evidence shown in the thermometer reading. The father paused, recognizing that this week was actually different, and that there was an understandable reason for the child's behavior.

Demonstrating Empathy

Understanding the child's perspective can help pave the way for empathy. One family had a son who attended a very high-pressure school. The parents wanted the son to work on homework in a common space in the house, rather than in his bedroom, because he was more efficient and focused when he worked in the common space. However, once they realized that their introverted son needed a break from people after a busy day at school, they were better able to understand why he wanted to go right to his room. This helped reduce conflict, and they were able to work on solutions together that would address everyone's concerns.

Empathy involves an understanding of why someone does something or feels a certain way. If caregivers can appreciate potential reasons for their child's behavior, then they will likely respond differently to their child. If their child comes home from school in a bad mood or with an "attitude," can they think of possible reasons for this? Might they have done poorly on an assignment? Had an argument with a friend? Just be really tired? You can empathize with the parent that it is hard to cope with a child who vents their frustrations on the parent. If the parent understands that their child's presentation likely has to do with other irritations, they may be able to respond in a less volatile manner.

Encourage parents to think of three to five reasons why their child might be behaving in a way that they do not prefer. Then ask them how they might respond differently, depending upon the reason.

Building Caregiver Conversation and Collaboration Skills

Avoid difficult conversations when they are unlikely to bring about a positive outcome. The parent can let the child know, when appropriate, that the child does not have to tell them information that they do not want to share. For example, a parent might say, "Sounds like you might have had a rough day at school. You don't have to tell me about it but if you want to, I am here." When parents decide to ask "What's wrong?" questions, prepare them for different child responses. If the child then says, "Yeah, I don't want to talk about it," the parent can just say, "Okay," and walk away, knowing that they are setting the stage for better interactions later. If the child tells them what happened, remind them not to go right into problem-solving mode if that is not what the child is looking for. Teach them some active listening, reflection, and validation skills if they are at a loss for how to respond. There may be times when it is important for the parent to know what happened or at least that something terrible did not happen. In these moments, the caregiver might say, "Taking care of serious things is part of my job as a parent. Just tell me the basics, so I know if I need to do something about this."

Healthy conversations can reduce conflict and begin the process of co-creating solutions to predictable and recurring problems, such as those around activities of daily living. Role playing conversations with parents can be a good way to start them on the road to better collaborations and conversations with their children. Let parents know that every interaction does not need to become a negotiation, but that positive conversations will allow for collaborations, problem solving, validating, and limit-setting.

Redirection

When parents predict that a negative behavior is about to occur or is starting, they can learn to direct the child's attention to something new, preventing the behavior from occurring or escalating. An example would be when a child starts walking toward a sibling, presumably to annoy them, and the parent says, "Hey, how about a snack?" Using redirection requires parents to intervene early with a shift away from inciting situations. Redirection can be especially helpful if it includes calming or relaxation techniques, such as those described by Goodyear-Brown (2021). Parents can think of it as hitting the "reset button."

Redirection is distinct from reward. As long as children are not rewarded by the redirection, this is a useful skill for parents to employ. Sometimes redirections or distractions, such as extra device use or snacks that are not usually permitted, can create problems by providing an incentive for threatening to misbehave.

Use Worksheet 15.3, "Building Skills," with parents to work on these skills.

Difficult Conversations with the Caregiver

Some information and observations lead to difficult conversations with the caregivers. Even when approaching a potentially charged conversation, you are still partnering with the parent. You are offering yourself as a team member, with everyone having essentially the same goal: improvement in the concerns that brought them in.

Communicating to the Caregiver the Need to Do Things Differently

One difficult topic that arises frequently with caregivers involves telling them that there are more helpful ways to parent than the way they have been going about it. Now, putting it that way, even couched in the language of this sentence, will likely be off-putting and sound judgmental. However, if you instead communicate that the child has significant needs, that their behaviors are really challenging, and that there are techniques the parents can use that will likely be more effective given their child's needs, you will go farther. The message is not that "you caused this behavior in your child" but that "the child's difficult behavior requires more tools in your toolkit. I can help give you those tools and teach you to use them."

Consider the following example scenario. A mother brings her 4-year-old child in for therapy. You complete your assessment and observe them interacting. You see that there are more effective ways that this mother could interact with her child that would improve the child's behavior. During the session, the child makes multiple attempts to get her mother's attention. Her mother focuses on the questions you are asking and does her best to ignore the child. The child eventually stops making overt social bids and instead starts throwing toys. One nearly hits the mother, who yells at the child to stop, without providing the desired attention or an alternative activity to occupy the child. The mother tells you that they have seen another clinician who told her it was her fault that her child acted that way.

You are thinking to yourself, "Yes, if you did things differently life would indeed be a lot easier for both of you." You choose not to say this to the mother directly. Instead, you say "Children come into the world with different temperaments. What works well for one child might not work as well for another. You let me know that your child is pretty energetic and kind of impulsive. That is challenging for any parent. It sure does not make parenting easy! I have some ideas that could help. Because your child is young, you will need to be involved in the work we do. I think you will be able to really make a difference with your child!"

As clinicians, we may identify a conversation that we want to have with a caregiver, or know would be helpful to have, that we anticipate will be difficult. The content may be uncomfortable for us, the parent may have a history of belligerent responses, or we may feel unsure of what wording to use. Worksheet 15.4, "What Is Getting in the Way of Having a Difficult Discussion with a Parent?" can help clarify the conversation you want to have with the parent, name barriers, and identify solutions.

A New Diagnosis for the Child

It is also possible that you have used your knowledge and clinical judgment to make a diagnosis that surprises the family. Your strategies for this conversation may include:

- Talking about the symptoms and how they match the parent's report of their own child.
- Informing them that this diagnosis is a name for what they already knew.
- Using the diagnosis to develop a treatment pathway.
- Discussing the normal grief parents have about new diagnoses.
- Discussing the reasons why and ways a diagnosis might change over time. Factors that will impact a changing presentation include development and growth, intervention and accommodations, and changes in settings and expectations.
- Remembering not to shy away from the discussion. Other professionals, such as oncologists, do not withhold diagnoses. We should not either.
- Allowing feelings to be present without immediately shifting away from them, validating them, and remembering them from one week to the next.

Many attributes and behaviors can decrease parental effectiveness. Hone in on what is getting in the way and how to address it. An awareness of challenging parental attributes is a first step to avoiding pitfalls, some of which we address in the next part.

WORKSHEET 15.1

Parent Values

- What values do I have as a parent?
- What is my view about the role of a parent?
- How did my parents raise me?
- What did my parents do well?
- What mistakes did they make?
- What is an ideal parent?
- In what ways would I hope to emulate my parents?
- How do I view the balance of supporting kids and building independence?
- What am I proud about in my parenting or in my time with my children in my family?
- What do I wish I had done differently?
- When families have different parenting values than I do, how do I manage it?
- How do I cope when other parents in my community have a difference of opinion?
- What do I get out of helping other people?
- Am I cooperative or competitive as a parent with others in the community?
- How would I rate these parenting values on a scale of not important to very important:

warmth	teaching
playing	building character
honesty	openness
rules	time together between parent and child
obedience	love
forgiveness	structure
clarity	discipline
achievement in school	preparing for college
preparing for a job/career	achievement in arts, sports, or music
being in an orchestra or on a team	following in parent's footsteps

WORKSHEET 15.2

Model of an Ideal Parent

Examples (real or fictional):

1. ____

2. ____

3. ____

Qualities that make them a good parent:

Ways that I can bring these qualities into my everyday life:

WORKSHEET 15.3

Building Skills

Self-awareness and recognizing what I say and do that makes the situation worse	
What can I do?	Observable goal(s)
Frustration tolerance	
What can I do?	Observable goal(s)
Lowering the thermostat and affect regulation	
What can I do?	Observable goal(s)
Perspective taking	
What can I do?	Observable goal(s)
Empathy	
What can I do?	Observable goal(s)
Conversation and collaboration skills	
What can I do?	Observable goal(s)
Validation	
What can I do?	Observable goal(s)

WORKSHEET 15.4

What Is Getting in the Way of Having a Difficult Discussion with a Parent?

- The difficult discussion I would like to have is ______________________________

  ____

  I feel this is important because ______________________________

  ____

- What worries do I have? ______________________________

  ____

  How can I address them? ______________________________

  ____

- How do I think the parent will respond? ______________________________

  ____

- How can I address that? ______________________________

  ____

- What are my thoughts or fears about what will happen? ______________________________

  ____

- How can I address those? ______________________________

  ____

- What else can I do to set the conversation up for success? ______________________________

  ____

- Who can help me think through these concerns? ______________________________

- When can I meet with the parent? ______________________________

PART VI

When Something Goes Wrong

Potential Pitfalls in Parent Guidance

Sometimes you watch a television show or a movie and think, "Why is the character doing that? That will not end well!" This part is intended to help avoid that scenario in our professional lives. There are many pitfalls that we encounter in parent coaching. Some are clinical; others are ethical and legal. We have all hit stuck points in treatment. In the following chapters, we address some of these perils and stuck points.

CHAPTER 16

Pitfalls with the Parent or with the Therapist

There are many ways a caregiver can present that makes parent guidance more challenging. We spell out some of the ways here and talk about ways to "partner," remembering the "P" in PACT, in order to effect positive change.

Addressing Pitfalls with the Parent: Dealing with a Challenging Caregiver

The Stonewall

The stonewall will not let you make any interventions. You know the stonewall by help-rejecting statements such as "We've already tried that," by their dismissive body language and facial expressions, or actively arguing with your advice. You find yourself frustrated and at a loss for what to recommend. This family came to you for help; you would like to help them but they will not let you. However, they remain in your office saying, "Help us," while simultaneously holding up a stop sign to your suggestions.

STRATEGY: *Get Over the Wall*

- Name the pattern.
- Identify potential reasons for the pattern.
- Instill hope.
- Use a paradoxical approach.

The first step to helping the stonewall parent is to name the pattern out loud. Caregivers then have the choice to recognize it or not. If you have a solid relationship with the parent, you might say something such as "Often you say [for example] that you already tried what I suggested and it did not work. Sometimes things need to be fine-tuned in order to work. Let's dig in, see what you have done, and see if it makes sense to try something similar, but with some tweaking." Alternatively, it might go something like "There seem to be some things getting in the way of trying the ideas we've talked about. Very often you say [for example], 'I already tried that and it didn't work.' We don't wind up moving forward. You have been working really hard in your parenting and things have not been changing much. You and your child deserve to have things going more smoothly. What can we do to make it easier to try some new ideas?" Or try the paradoxical approach: "You seem to have tried most of my suggestions. It's got to be frustrating that the usual suggestions have not worked for you. Is it worth looking at them again and trying to figure out what's happening? Or should we leave that problem as is and focus on something else?"

There are many reasons why parents may adopt a stonewall stance. Maybe they feel defeated. Perhaps there is a desire for a "magical" solution that requires no effort. Maybe they feel embarrassed or defensive. Maybe they cannot let go of the idea that their child should be different than they are. Getting to the bottom of it will help you determine how to manage it. If they feel defeated, instill hope. Let them know that, in your experience, other families have made changes with these techniques. Do some cheerleading. You can be intense and dramatic, if that is your style. Look them in the eye and let them know that you are in this with them. If they feel embarrassed or defensive, be gentle and validating. Remind them that what they have been trying has not been working and, if they can rally their efforts, they will see positive outcomes.

Another useful way to approach this type of parent is to talk about what constitutes good parent guidance, and that they are worthy of and entitled to quality treatment. You could say something such as "We can sit here cataloging and rejecting ideas to try but that is not good therapy. I want to try and be the best therapist I can for you, and I value your time. Let's see what we can do to make this the most effective therapy we can, so that things are better for your child and for you. They deserve it and so do you."

You might also say, "I know that this takes a lot of energy. It is really hard work. And you do not even know that it will work. For the moment, I will hold the hope and know that it can work. That will be part of my job. And then I will work with you to figure out how to give it a try. I just ask that you trust me enough to give it a try."

The Wile E. Coyote

The parent we have dubbed the Wile E. Coyote parent does the same ineffective thing over and over, despite seemingly earnest attempts to help their child. They are likely unaware that they are making the same mistake repeatedly. They may feel that they are trying; in fact trying hard. But while they are putting a lot of energy in, they are doing so inflexibly. An example is the parent who sets bedtime at 8:00 P.M. every night, tells the child to go off to bed, and expects them to obey. They do not change their strategy, despite the reality that their child screams as soon as it is bedtime and does not go to sleep until after midnight.

STRATEGY: *Build Flexibility*

- Help the caregiver understand that they are repeating unhelpful efforts. Help them recognize the pattern and understand that with some potentially small shifts their energy expenditure will be much more fruitful. However, without those shifts the Road Runner (their child) will get around their traps every time.
- Use language such as "unhelpful" and "not working," rather than "good," "bad," or other terms that sound evaluative. Focus on what is observable.
- Inoculate the parent. Make certain that they know that there will be increased energy expenditure initially. Stepping out of habits is challenging. Doing anything contrary to one's habits or one's intuition is, by definition, harder. However, let them know that the initial outlay of effort will pay off in the long term, with interactions requiring less energy and life becoming easier.

The Wet Noodle

The parent we call the wet noodle is the powerless parent. They might fear that any change could make things even worse. They feel too helpless or afraid to make any demands on their child, who may have enormous tantrums when they do. Philosophically, they may believe that they should allow their child a fully unfettered life experience, one that inspires exploration. They may lack the skills to figure out how to set limits. This type of parent may have grown up in a cruel household and, to them, any limit setting feels abusive. There are many possible reasons for why a parent would be reluctant to implement rules, create boundaries, or make demands. It is worth noting that there is support in the psychological literature for the authoritative parenting style characterized by both warmth and structure. A limit-setting style has been associated with social competence in toddlers (Houck & LeCuyer-Maus, 2002), and the authoritative parenting style has been linked to increased psychosocial competence and fewer behavioral concerns in adolescence (Lamborn et al., 1991), and better life satisfaction in adolescents and young adults (Lavric & Naterer, 2020). Developing skills and behaviors consistent with the authoritative parenting style is seen in Kazdin's (2008) work and in parent–child interaction therapy (PCIT; Zisser & Eyberg, 2010). For some caregivers, teaching them skills alone will allow them to improve their ability to set limits. Others will need more, such as addressing family-of-origin issues, coping with feelings of rejection when their child gets angry at them, and troubleshooting their concerns robustly.

STRATEGY: *Strengthen the Parent*

- Determine the underlying issue leading to discomfort with limit setting and address it directly.
- Educate the caregiver about the role of parents in the family and the benefit of structure for children.
- Identify the caregiver's values and link them to parenting behaviors.
- Identify the characteristics that the caregiver hopes their child will demonstrate

and ascertain whether their current parenting style will help the child to develop them.

Figure out why this parent is struggling with setting limits. Work on the underlying issue, whether it is their experience with their family of origin, their understanding of what will allow a child to flourish, or the backlash that they expect to receive from their child or the community. Do psychoeducation about the benefits of structure for children. Teach strategies for optimal parenting and responding to difficult behavior. Shore them up by reminding them of the competence they feel in other situations outside of parenting. Sometimes it helps for parents to know that raising children can be very humbling for most people. Cheerlead when they make small changes. Help them recognize and celebrate their successes.

If enforcing family rules feels abusive to caregivers, elucidate the differences and help them understand that setting limits, creating structure, and making demands are important aspects of parenting. If their parents were abusive or overly permissive, talk about the hard job of learning what it is to be a skilled parent. Brainstorm with them about the role of a parent. Talk about what qualities they hope their children develop as they grow older and what it will take to get them there. Help the caregivers shift from being a wet noodle to being a firm and loving force in their child's life.

Many caregivers do not have a model for setting limits beyond rewards and punishments, despite the clear benefits of limit setting for children (Denham et al., 2000). The wet noodle has particular trouble with saying no to their children or setting appropriate limits and rules. Providing explanations for children about what can and cannot happen is a natural way to build in more thoughtful limits for all caregivers. For example, "We aren't having ice cream today because we plan to go to the ice cream shop on Friday." Gary Landreth, a pioneer in child-centered psychotherapy, developed a limit-setting approach (2002) that works well and instills responsibility. For example, if a child is kicking a toy truck, the approach might be:

1. State the rule: "Trucks are not for kicking."
2. Provide an alternative: "Balls are for kicking" or "Trucks are for pushing."
3. Build responsibility: "If you choose to keep kicking the truck, the truck will have to go away for today."

The consequence built into the last step is within the child's power to change, if it is possible for the child to manage the impulse. This is a set routine that parents, especially those who describe themselves as egalitarian and who sometimes dislike setting rules, may be able to adopt.

The Control Freak

The control freak does not feel comfortable giving their child reasonable freedoms, as they are certain that their way is the right way. Their goal in seeking treatment is often to find ways to make their children conform to their restrictions rather than changing their own behavior or viewpoint. Despite seeking treatment, they are not looking to make change. Potential reasons for controlling behavior include anxiety about their child failing, being hurt, or being embarrassed. For some caregivers, they feel that if they manage their children closely enough, then these unpleasant experiences do not have to happen.

STRATEGY: *Help Them Loosen the Reins*

- Empathize with the aspects of parenting that are hard for this parent, namely wanting to oversee many aspects of their child's life so that the child either will not fail in any endeavor or will be very successful in life.
- Focus on independence and responsibility, along with ways to foster these important attributes.
- Provide some space for the parent to express their feelings when, for example, their child messes up.

Acknowledge how hard it is to not have continual feedback about their child's activities or to let their children fail. Would that parents could wrap their children in metaphorical bubble wrap and never have anything bad happen to them. Work with caregivers to understand the benefits, to both the child and to their relationship with the child, of giving up some control. Provide space for the parent to talk about the difficulties in letting children make their own mistakes and help them recognize the benefits of children learning independence skills.

The Martyr

The martyr parent uses therapy to impress on you the depth of their suffering and struggle with their child as well as the nobility in their parenting. It may even seem that they choose situations that will lead to pain and hardship. They may seem beleaguered. It can be challenging to move parents out of the martyrdom role, especially if they find a part of it gratifying.

STRATEGY: *Help the Parent Take Charge for Their Child and Themself*

- Acknowledge the parent's desire to help their child and that this determined willingness to help their child is a strength to be used in treatment.
- Recognize, with the caregiver, that parenting is challenging and that even the most difficult aspects cannot be avoided.
- Identify together concrete steps they can take to help their child.
- Anticipate and help process the feelings that they may have or develop during the time you work together.

Find out why the parents got into this role. Will it be a loss to them in some way to move out of the martyr position? Are they similar to the other challenging parents we have discussed, such as the "wet noodle" or the "Wile E. Coyote"? Help parents commit to more effective parenting, using motivational strategies. Note that the effort they put in will pay off in the long run. This strategy utilizes the strength of this style, which is the determined willingness to help their child. Remind them that they are the most important person in their child's life and what a crucial role they play in their child's development. With this knowledge, they may seek less validation for their suffering and struggles and be able to move toward effective parenting.

The Negative Nelly: The Angry or Sad Parent

The parent who has nothing positive to say about their child and may just want to share a list of grievances is hard to tolerate. Anger, sadness, or resentment may pervade the sessions with them. This affect overwhelms the session and interferes with progress. The apparent intention is to get you to validate their righteous anger and belief that it is the child who is in the wrong. Think about how you can listen to and validate their experience without reinforcing entrenchment in the current modes of interacting and feeling. What tools can you use to alter the dynamic so that you are able to move forward?

STRATEGY: *Locate the Problem*

- Ascertain whether the problem is the caregiver's more general negative style or whether it is specific to the relationship with the child.
- If it is a more general negative style, gently address how it might be impacting the child and talk about whether you can work with the caregiver on this issue or whether individual psychotherapy focused on the cause, for example, depression, is warranted.
- If it is a relational issue, use the relationship-building strategies discussed elsewhere in this book (see Chapter 14).

This requires careful differential diagnosis. Does the pervasive affect reside in the caregiver or in the relationship with the child? If the caregiver generally presents this way, determine whether parent coaching is adequate or whether individual psychotherapy, either initially on its own or in conjunction with parent coaching, is needed. If the negativity is focused primarily on the child, then direct efforts at improving the relationship between the caregiver and the child. Help the caregiver adjust their viewpoint such that, even if the child is primarily at fault for difficult interactions, the parent can be the genesis of change for the child and the relationship. Start with our more basic strategies such as child-led play and building conversation skills.

Looking in the Mirror: Pitfalls with the Therapist That Undermine Our Effectiveness

Some challenges or pitfalls have to do with assumptions, or our stance—the way we, as therapists, approach our clients. In this section we discuss the challenges that can negatively affect the thoughtful and considered work we do.

The Therapist as Friend

You may be in this pitfall if you imagine becoming a friend to the parent or if the parent makes comments to suggest that is how they see you. It is a hard balance to strike between sharing instructive stories and being so friendly that the therapy devolves into overly familiar conversation. Behaving in an overly friendly way might seem to be the antidote, but it can cause other problems. When parents feel more comfortable taking advice from a friend than from a professional, this feels more like a benefit than a pitfall. However, when the parents see us as friends, our skilled stance is jeopardized, and it may be harder for parents to take the neutral advice we do have to offer.

We can also become tired and "run out of steam." With patients whom we like, it might be tempting to seek support or validation from them. They may also enjoy this favored role over the more vulnerable "patient" position. When you recognize this dynamic in yourself or in the parents you are working with, remember that despite the fact that it may feel right, befriending a patient is a barrier to effective parent guidance and jeopardizes treatment effectiveness.

STRATEGY: *Be Professional*

When you recognize your desire to befriend patients, or have a relationship outside of therapy, remember your professional role. This may be a time to seek your own therapy or expand your own friendship group. It may be a sign of burnout. If you have the distortion that this parent is "uniquely" matched to be your friend, remind yourself that the context in which you met them prohibits this shift and will damage their treatment. Seek support through colleagues, consultation, or supervision.

If the parent is seeking to be friends with you, discuss this fact explicitly. Acknowledge that the therapist–patient relationship is an unusual and one-sided one, but because it is one-sided, it serves to help them. What we do in therapy is not about engaging in typical interaction patterns. If therapists interact with clients as friends and acquaintances interact with them in everyday situations, there would be no benefit to coming to therapy. When you notice that therapy time is shifting away from the parents and toward you or shared interests, make these detours short, unless they have specific therapeutic value, and turn back to your mission of helping them with parenting.

The Wayward Therapist

There are many ways in which we can lose our therapy direction. When you notice that you are no longer focused on helping to improve parenting, you are in this pitfall. Chatting about other topics briefly might serve to improve rapport. When these off-topic conversations take significant time away from therapeutic interventions, you need to find the path back to your shared objectives.

STRATEGY: *Refocus*

When you identify this pitfall, ask yourself why you are engaging in this behavior. Is something going on in your own life? Are you unsure of what to do to be helpful?

Do the caregivers seem comfortable chatting, which avoids the hard work of moving toward change? Do you need peer consultation or supervision to return to more therapeutic activities? Are you engaging in this behavior for their benefit or for yours?

Watch how the patient is responding. Is it reinforcing to have their attention and admiration? If they are more comfortable in session, is it because it feels like a conversation with a friend, rather than a therapeutic endeavor? If they appear less comfortable, is it because they prefer to return to the more useful conversation of changing their own or their child's behavior? The key to avoiding this pitfall is to retain the focus and direction of the parent guidance, even when we are fatigued or losing sight of the goal, or when patients enjoy our off-topic wanderings.

We may fall into this trap because we are feeling lost and directionless. Return to the presenting problem, your treatment plan, and access to supervision and consultation for direction. Consider the goals you have identified with the family and reflect on your own barriers to change in order to get back on track.

The Therapist as Johnny One-Note (or Johnny One-Manual)

Some clinicians or treatment programs use a single method to treat all patients. This can be very effective when targeting one specific disorder that responds well to a research-documented protocol. If you have the opportunity to attain specialized training in evidence-based treatment protocols, take advantage of it. There are risks, however, in only having a hammer when not everything is a nail. Some clinicians continue to try the same interventions repeatedly, or apply the same interventions across the board, even when they are not achieving success. Be wary of "blaming" the parent who does not progress when you have not adapted your approach to their needs.

STRATEGY: *Continually Assess the Appropriateness of the Approach and Progress*

Each parent who comes to therapy has the right to an approach that is based on evidence that it will be successful and, at the same time, is individualized to their needs. If you have a "preferred" intervention approach, inform parents at the beginning of the treatment that you utilize that approach. If the patient is not making progress with that approach, either change your strategy or refer to them to clinicians who can offer them other options. All parent guidance requires consistent monitoring of progress and adaptation based on whether the client is making progress or not. Most clinicians, even those primarily wedded to one approach, have a few other tools to use when they are not seeing improvements. Keep abreast of new literature and strategies concerning parent guidance in order to continue growing as an expert.

CASE STUDY: The One-Diagnosis Therapist

A family brought their daughter to therapy. The child had behaviors consistent with a trauma reaction. The therapist met with the daughter for individual therapy and provided guidance to the parents. This therapist had recently become trained in attention-deficit/hyperactivity disorder (ADHD) treatment and its different presentation in females as compared to males. She diagnosed the girl with ADHD and provided guidance to the parents that targeted improving attention and building executive function skills, seemingly ignoring the trauma symptoms and other behaviors that were inconsistent with the girl's ADHD diagnosis. The therapist persevered with her approach even though there was no clear improvement. When the clinician moved to a new state, the child and her parents were transferred to a new therapist who focused on the child's presenting complaint of trauma. With individual psychotherapy, psychoeducation, and parent guidance focused on trauma, the girl and her parents were able to ameliorate the effects of the trauma. The secondary attentional symptoms improved significantly as well.

The Therapist as a Runaway Train

Another reason a therapist might continue on a path that is not helping the child and parents to make progress is that the clinician is comfortable continuing with the plan they began, has difficulty switching gears, or lacks alternatives, like the "Johnny one-note" therapist we discussed earlier. Or perhaps the strategy is the best practice for a specific diagnosis but may not be working for this individual, or the referral source or the caregiver asked for a particular treatment approach. Keeping a parent in treatment when there is no clear benefit or path for increasing effectiveness is an ethical concern. Do not continue using the same strategy as if time is all that is needed to make a difference. Just because you've become stuck does not mean that you have to stop treatment; it means that you must think about what might be helpful to get the therapy unstuck.

STRATEGY: *Take a Different Track*

Part of assessing treatment efficacy is talking to the parents and gaining their perspective about what is working and what is not. How would you know, and how would they know, if you were progressing? Are they getting closer to achieving their goals? We are not suggesting that you try a different technique each week just because you recently learned something new. We are suggesting an intentional approach to change with well-thought-out strategies, a regular assessment of progress, and adaptation based on results.

We ask parents to try interventions in between sessions and to let us know how they went. We may ask them to gather data on their efforts to then review with us at the next session. When they do bring us the report about the intervention or the child's behavior, we can use it to cheer them on or fine-tune or adjust the plan. If they did not follow through on the data collection or intervention, we can determine what the barriers are. There may be practical barriers to what we devised, or maybe they did not agree with or understand the recommendation. If you try the same "homework" several weeks in a row and it does not get implemented, it is worth figuring out why that might be. Even if you believe that this is the best intervention for this family and this problem, it cannot work if it is not implemented. Say something like "We have talked about this piece of homework for several weeks, and it is not happening. Let's talk about why and whether it makes sense to keep trying this homework or to try something else."

The Therapist's Feelings Are Getting in the Way

As a therapist, your feelings toward the parents will be valuable data that can either help or hinder the treatment. We gain important data about the patients, and perhaps ourselves, by reflecting on our responses to and feelings about them. There are a range of feelings that you may have. For example, you may find yourself feeling frustrated or saddened when caregivers do not follow recommendations, or you may feel angry if the children suffer because of the caregiver's choices and behavior. Sometimes an acknowledgment by colleagues of the hard work you are doing can help to return feelings to a more productive range. For some therapists, it feels harder to work with parents than with children. Intense feelings about the parents may signal that you need to find empathy for the caregivers, or that you need to step back and check whether there is a concrete problem getting in the way of the therapeutic interventions.

Difficulty stems from reactions that are not recognized and addressed. If you are frustrated, it is easier to elicit empathy when you recognize your own feelings and try to understand why the caregivers are behaving the way they are.

STRATEGY: *Recognize and Manage Your Feelings*

When you are having stronger feelings about the parents than you typically do, it is time to get consultation or supervision. Use colleagues and supervisors to support you in your work. Whatever the response you have, recognize it as helpful clinical information. Perhaps others have similar feelings about this parent, which may be useful feedback. As you recognize your own feelings, they can guide you regarding how to be more helpful. When you are with the caregiver, do not communicate anger or frustration. Focus on the reasons why they are behaving as they are, which will help you empathize with them and continue to work productively.

The Therapist Is Competitive with the Caregiver

You may recognize this pitfall when you feel competitive with the parent about the child's connection to you, when you compare the child client to your own children, when you feel smug about how great you are at parenting, or when the parent makes comments about your superiority or negative judgments. The therapist also may "show off" about either their superior therapeutic skills or showcase how well their own child is doing. Listen for statements by the parent that suggest you are dealing with this pitfall. For example, parents may make comments about how you would handle a situation at home, such as "I'd like to see you handle it when he destroys your favorite mug." They may also hint that you do not understand the level of difficulty in parenting this child, with statements like "you should take him home for the weekend."

Caregivers may also suggest that they believe you are superior, with comments such as "I wish I could think of saying it like you do." This pitfall is a barrier to parent guidance because it can disempower the parent, undermine the alliance, and limit the parents' ability to see themself as a proactive and powerful agent for change in their child.

STRATEGY: *Keep Your Eyes on the Goal*

If you are feeling superior to the parent, remind yourself that the goal of the therapy is for the child to feel and behave better with the parent, not with you. When you are tempted to make a self-disclosure about your parenting successes, consider why you are doing it and whether it will be helpful to the therapeutic process moving forward. If you choose to self-disclose, keep it brief and focused on what will be therapeutic. Do not turn the conversation to yourself.

When you notice that the caregivers are making comments that point to this pitfall, acknowledge the difficulty they are experiencing, their unique situation, their effort toward solving it (including by seeing you), and your belief in their ability to effect change. Provide hope by referring to your experience working with other parents, while acknowledging the challenge of living with difficult behavior full time.

The Therapist as Judge

You may be dealing with this pitfall when the parent says, "You're going to say I did this wrong but . . ." You may also find yourself feeling judgmental about the parent, given that they make some repeated "errors" or do not adequately follow through on agreed-upon interventions. The parents may also be judging themselves when they fall short of their own hopes or expectations. Parents sometimes "confess" their poor behavior in order to attain your absolution, which can be an unhealthy dynamic that may serve to sustain rather than change those behaviors.

STRATEGY: *Recognize That This Is Not a Trial*

Help the parent focus on your shared aim of providing more effective parenting. Rather than judging, together examine the helpfulness of different strategies. You, the therapist, are an equally responsible teammate rather than an arbiter of good and bad parenting. Parents also benefit from reminders that parents are people too. They cannot follow through on the "perfect" thing to do or say each time and, because you know this, you are not judging them. When you look, with parents, at the barriers to behaving as they wish to, it can reduce negative self-evaluations and increase comfort in talking about foibles, creating a smoother pathway to change. If the parents judge themselves too harshly, overfocusing on their problems as parents, encourage them to turn their attention to parenting successes and the positive steps they are taking toward change. It is likely that there have been positive moments with their children during which they believe they have done well. Help them bring those moments into the session as well.

When a caregiver starts "confessing," as just described, it is useful to validate their admission. However, if you notice that a pattern of judging themselves too harshly recurs frequently, to no therapeutic end, know that it may be sustaining the behavior and stalling progress. In this scenario, it is worth stating something like "It's really hard to put into practice the things we talk about. I am concerned that we are getting stuck focusing on what did not go well rather than on figuring out how to move forward. Let's try to figure out what got in the way of doing what you had planned, or hoped, to do."

The Family Calls You Out on a Mistake

When families let us know that we made a mistake, we have the opportunity to rectify it. We are fortunate when they do. The alternative is that they feel less comfortable with us, making it likely that our work will be less effective.

Sometimes we do not feel that we made an error. At other times we agree that our suggestion was problematic or that we made some other mistake. Either way, the family believes that we did, and we need to respond in a helpful way. We are human and we will make mistakes or interact in a way that makes the parent feel uncomfortable. Some such situations are unavoidable. Unavoidable mistakes might include running late to a session because we are dealing with a crisis or being away on vacation when a family is coping with a significant stressor. Some mistakes might be avoidable, such as missing an appointment because we forgot or double-booked. We hope this sort of thing never happens, but it does.

STRATEGY: *Own It*

It is important to acknowledge when we make mistakes. Though it may be difficult, try not to be defensive. This is helpful behavior to model with parents for use with their children. Also, being vulnerable can make us more approachable. If you did make an error, apologize for it. Do what you can to rectify it.

If you do not feel that you made an error, try to understand why the family thinks you did, recognizing the kernel of truth that you can. You may talk about how you work and why a similar matter may or may not come up again. Let the parent know that it is important that they tell you when they have concerns so that you can talk about them openly, even when you approach them from a different perspective.

There are times when a caregiver is upset, not because you made an error, but because they were struggling and you were unable to solve the problem. This is the case in the example of being on vacation when a crisis happens for a family. They understand that it is reasonable for you to take a vacation. They also are aware of the structures in place to support them while you are away. That may not keep them from feeling hurt, let down, unsupported, or jealous of the better life that they imagine you have. The family knows that this is not a mistake that you made, but they may have the affective experience that needs to be addressed in moving forward with your parenting intervention.

The purpose of this chapter is to help you recognize that there are ways to be mindful of potential pitfalls in parent guidance. As always, being intentional will help. Prevent problems by thinking through who your patient is, by deciding how you intend to tackle the issues presented, and by guiding sessions in a structured and boundaried manner. In the next chapter, we discuss the related topic of difficulties that arise in the therapeutic process.

CHAPTER 17

Pitfalls in the Therapeutic Process

Pitfalls and stuck points come up in the process of therapy. There are a multitude of factors that interfere with the therapeutic process. Identifying the specific problems will assist you in overcoming them. Use Worksheet 17.1, "In My Parent Guidance Work I Am Struggling with . . ." to help think through this process.

Differing Philosophies

Should children behave? This question is more complex than it seems and is often at the heart of caregiver disagreements. Are children in need of clear direction from parents, or should they be setting their own agendas from early on? To what degree should parents control their children's paths? What does raising a well-behaved child mean in terms of the child developing into an assertive, thoughtful, and independent adult? Although there is no treatment protocol that we know of that requires considering these issues, we think it is a useful exercise. Answers to these questions feel so basic that they become unexamined assumptions.

Taken from philosophy, dialectics is defined as a system of reasoning whereby two seemingly opposing circumstances can both be true. This concept applies to parent guidance work—for example, Miller and colleagues (2002) note the dialectic of accepting the adolescent client as they are and also expecting change when working with adolescent clients. Similarly, in parent guidance you accept the parent as they are and also work with them toward change. At the same time, you encourage the parents to accept their child as they are and also help the child change.

Managing Differing Philosophies: Yours and Theirs

Your delivery of parent guidance may be influenced by your personal beliefs and philosophy on childrearing. You have ideas, based on your training and life experience, about how parenting should be done. Similarly, parents have a philosophy about parenting that is rooted in a temporal and cultural context. When there is a difference in philosophies, step back and ask yourself if your belief is grounded in psychological research or in the way you were raised and the culture you live in. You may also help parents step back and evaluate whether their philosophical difference with you is based on important, deeply held values, or simply a habitual way of doing things. Think about the ways your philosophy influences the work you do, whether it is critical to hold to, or whether it too should be placed in a sociocultural and temporal context.

Parents benefit from new ways to think about parenting, but as long as what the caregivers are doing is not abusive or neglectful, you have the difficult task of recognizing that parenting decisions are theirs and not yours. Letting go of parenting control can be hard for therapists when caregivers make decisions that the therapist would not. It is important to remember that, despite philosophical mismatches, you have helpful strategies to offer.

STRATEGY: *Accept the Limitations of Your Role and Don't Debate*

Your job is not to get the family to function as you would like them to. It is to help them reach their objectives. When there is a mismatch, the first step is to accept the family's style and continue. Conversations should focus on what is likely to be effective in addressing the issues that bring them to your office. This is not a time to get into a debate about which approach is "better." An obvious example may be physical punishment. A parent may lightly slap the hand of a young child after they hit a sibling. We can talk about what our professions recommend, what has been found to be helpful, and how we can work to develop other ways of managing difficult behavior. It would not be helpful to engage in a belabored lecture or debate the merits of our philosophy of discipline.

Another example that comes up in clinical practice involves working with children of immigrant parents. Parents raised in other cultures may have practices that are different from what are typically seen in the United States, leading to mismatches with not only the therapist, but also with the larger community in which they live. Acknowledge this difficulty and recognize, with them, the realities of the situation. Ask what differences they see. What are the most important parenting concerns to them and why? Answers to these questions will clarify mismatches and allow for intentional choices about the focus of treatment.

Ambivalence within a Caregiver about How to Parent

Parenting is full of dialectics, including the dialectic of developing one of the closest relationships between two people, that of caregiver and child, and also expecting the caregiver to foster independence in this same child. Miller et al. (2002) refer to several additional dialectical parenting dilemmas that have been discussed in the literature, including leniency versus control and "normalizing pathological behavior and pathologizing normative behavior (p. 572)," to name a few. Others include children wanting independence and also needing parental support, and caregivers not wanting to be harsh with their children and also needing to provide consequences and limits. Parents are naturally expected to thread these needles. With your support, parents recognize that these dichotomies create dilemmas in making moment-to-moment parenting decisions. Whether it be seemingly opposing ideas or uncertainty about how a person wants to parent, honing in on what the parent values allows for forward movement.

STRATEGY: *Identify Values*

Step back and identify important values for this caregiver. Figure out how they would like to parent and what qualities they hope to instill in their child. Are the values reasonable for the whole family? If so, operationalize how to parent in accordance with those values. Without that exploration, treatment may not target the most important areas for change.

Differing Philosophies among Co-Parents

We encounter co-parents and other family units who are not unified in their view of child rearing. Your role, when they do not agree, is to help them come to a shared understanding of how they will parent, without taking sides. Guide each of them to articulate what is important to them, including how a child should behave, qualities they want to instill, and what parenting values they hold. It is tempting to side with the parent who you view as "right" or "closer to right." When you take sides, you lose the objectivity that helps both parents improve their parenting. It embeds you in their conflict, rather than letting you be someone who joins with both.

The potential pitfall here lies in not recognizing the divergent points of view, the dialectical dilemmas, the subjectivity in parenting, and the impossibility of doing parenting perfectly. What can occur is a caregiver who clings tightly to one part of the dialectic without seeing ways to become more balanced in their view, even if getting the ideal balance is not possible. Hopefully you, as the therapist, are not holding fast to the other side of the dialectic and in equally rigid ways pushing change.

We have seen different members of the caregiving team hold very different beliefs about how a child should be treated. Some parents become more polarized in their behavior toward the child very much in opposition to another parent's point of view. Maybe one parent thinks that there should be more leniency about a certain behavior, while another thinks that there should be very clear consequences for the same behavior. Parents may find that they are actually behaving in a way that is more polarized than they would normally choose, but feel they have to counter the other parent's strictness or leniency. While they are perhaps not fully comfortable in their stance, they each may feel stuck in this dynamic.

STRATEGY: *Move to the Middle*

If you are working with more than one caregiver, assess the ways they are and are not on the same page with each other. When there are mismatches between them, make them explicit for yourself and, depending upon the situation, for the parents too, so that they can be addressed and removed as treatment barriers. It is reasonable to consider whether the strategies that you are recommending are workable for all of the caregivers.

Teach the concept of dialectics and underscore the value of having multiple views. Highlight the dilemma, validate why it is challenging, and work with the parent or parents to find "the middle path" (Miller et al., 2007). For example, one parent might feel that the other is overbearing and therefore feel the need to be very hands off. The other parent feels that the first is too laissez-faire and that children need firm guidance. Both parents have tried a strategy that they perceive as "different" because the other parent is doing something else. Each parent is reacting to the perceived mistakes of the other, rather than charting their own natural course. Point out their behavior, as well as how it developed as a more polarized extreme version of what they would value, and ask whether they feel that embodying the extreme is what they want to do. This helps each of them to move to the middle or to find a compromise that they both can live with. Return to discussions about parenting values and how to achieve a less polarized stance. Have them imagine what that parenting behavior would look like.

Dynamics That Get in the Way of Moving Forward

Parents Are Not a Functioning Team

Caregivers may hold divergent views and still be effective co-parents. Demonstrating variety in approaches, styles, and skills in parenting can be helpful to children. In more collaborative dyads, parents can use these differences to their advantage, recognizing which tasks and interactions one parent will be effective with versus the other.

When caregivers are not functioning well as a team, differences are not strategically utilized and instead impede effectiveness. You may know they are in this situation when a parent reports how much easier being with the child was when the other parent was away. They may state that the child takes advantage of their disagreements or may be distressed by the observed conflict between them. Most clinicians who have been doing child and family work for any significant length of time have had at least one parent, if not both in a couple, talk to them, in ostensibly secret conversations, about the other parent's poor parenting. Remain neutral in the face of these "tattling" moments, as the effort to join with you works against having them function together more successfully.

STRATEGY: *Find the Kernel You Can Support*

Identify where each parent's skills lie and encourage them to be strategic about using them. If you are working with two parents and the behavior of neither one is reportable to child protective services, work to find the kernel of behavior in the less-skilled parent that you can support if there is one. Use this starting point to build momentum for adding more skills for both parents as time goes on.

Ideally parents will find strategies that they can agree to try. Start with the "low-hanging fruit" of a problem that is easier to solve. If you can find a first step that combines both of their ideas, this strategy may be more effective. The more specific and clear the solution is, the more likely it is that the parents will try it without reverting to old patterns. An example may be that one parent thinks a child should help with laundry and the other parent feels that the child is already busy enough. If they agree that asking the child to bring the laundry downstairs involves the child in the task but is not too taxing then that is a place to start.

Sometimes finding mutually agreed-upon strategies is difficult. Take, for example, the situation of a child who is being raised by a father and a stepmother. The stepmother has her own biological children, and the couple together has a biological child. The father and the stepmother do not agree on rules, especially for the identified patient, Jane. Jane believes she is being treated differently than the stepmother's biological children. Since the father works full-time, the stepmother is home more often with Jane and does the bulk of the parenting. The father brings the child in for therapy and has parenting sessions without the stepmother, who declines to be involved in therapy. The father is uncomfortable with how the stepmother parents Jane, but does not want to rock the boat with his new wife. This situation will take careful navigating and potentially challenging conversations with the father, who will have to take into account the stepmother's perspective, Jane's perspective, and the dynamics of the household in order to help the child.

The COW (Crisis Of the Week)

Unlike the elephant in the room, which does not get talked about, the COW in the room is constantly being talked about. A COW, or crisis of the week, presents readily during parent coaching because each week situations occur that seem pressing. These frequent issues, concerns, and crises may seem relevant to the work you are doing, but they can derail the ongoing process. For example, let us say you are working with parents on bedtime routines. The parents come into their next session and immediately tell you that their child got a terrible report card. You realize that 30 minutes have gone by, and you have not checked in about the bedtime routine.

You can recognize this pitfall when, instead of progressing toward the established treatment goal, each week a new, seemingly novel problem arises that takes up all of the airspace. During multiple sessions you realize that the parents are venting about the current stressor, which may be very legitimate, but you have not progressed toward the goals established on your treatment plan.

STRATEGY: *"Mooove" the COW*

There are multiple ways you can address the COW concern. Start by validating that the caregivers are coping with many stressors. They are probably unaware of the ways in which the COW interferes with progressing toward the goals they have set. Have an intentional dialogue about how much time to spend on new issues or crises versus staying on target with their therapeutic goals. If there are concrete problems that need solving, think about how to go about dealing with them. Is it a matter of referring the family to someone with more of a case management role or another service? If so, you can talk to the family about that referral and then you can focus on what brought them into therapy.

If the COWs do not require additional intervention, you may wonder why each session starts with one. If venting is getting in the way of therapeutic work, discuss its importance and value to the parents. Most people are unaware of the time they spend on different topics each week. Talk to them about designating time to discuss the current stressor and then making sure to spend the bulk of the time on the ongoing therapeutic interventions. Many people do well with a structured session. You can allot the first 10 or so minutes to current concerns and then move on to the ongoing work. Do not be rigid. Instead, gently remind the parents when they come in that you want to discuss what is on their mind currently for 10 minutes, and then to shift gears to what issue originally brought them in. After those 10 minutes, you can say, "Does this seem like a good time to move on to other things?"

You're Not Sure Where You Are Going: Do You Have a Therapeutic Contract?

There are times in your work with families that you feel like you are working harder than they are. They are coming in, or are not coming in, the time goes by, and they may not be following through on the tasks you discussed in treatment sessions. It is not clear that you and the parent are working toward the same goals. You may have a goal in mind, and it may even be one that you discussed together when creating or reviewing a treatment plan. However, either those goals, or how you intend to reach them, do not seem to be at the forefront for the family.

STRATEGY: *Time to Review*

What may be useful in this scenario is to go back to the metaphorical "therapeutic contract." This agreement is not a formal written contract that all parties sign; rather it is a shared understanding of what you are doing together. Ask yourself whether you have that therapeutic contract. Do you share the same goals and understanding about how to reach them? Hearken back to that shared understanding and perhaps review the treatment plan.

Maybe what the caregivers articulated as important to them early in treatment has changed. Perhaps refocusing on the goals will help them to summon the energy toward achieving them. If the parents do not agree with you about the goals, or cannot seem to generate energy towards achieving them, find out why. This is a time to say to them that you would like to review the goals to make sure everyone is on the same page. You want to ensure that you are being helpful to them, making good use of their time and efforts. Motivational interviewing (Miller & Rollnick, 2013) techniques may be useful here. It may be that they do share the goals, but are not ready to do what it would take to achieve them. If that is the case, and motivational interviewing or other techniques have not helped, then perhaps talk about other, more realistic goals. Return to goal setting and reviewing at any point when it seems helpful. Worksheet 17.2, "Parent Guidance Pitfalls Check-In," lists the pitfalls that we have discussed so far in this part of the book and offers a worksheet to help caregivers think through how they wish to proceed.

What to Watch for When Providing Parent Guidance Along with Child Therapy

Often the child is the patient, the person whom you are hoping to get to a better level of functioning. Sometimes in parent guidance the primary work is with the caregiver, and the therapist does no or little direct work with the child. If you start treatment with the child and then engage in parent guidance as a part of that treatment, you must continue to maintain a strong relationship with the child. In this scenario, you are helping the parent to change so that they can be more helpful to the child. When seeing both the child and the parent for guidance, avoid being seen as siding with the parent.

Depending on the age and developmental level of the child, talk with the child about the work you are doing with their caregiver. You should have a general conversation about the reason that you will be meeting with their caregiver, namely, to help them be more helpful to their child.

Also avoid joining with the child over the parent. some of this is inevitable, however. You are an adult that the child sees as supportive to them. EB has been reported by her teen clients to have endorsed numerous tattoos, piercings, and rights around drinking and marijuana over the years despite being a real square who does not advocate for any of these practices! Sometimes the therapist finds that the child told the parent that the therapist said this or that and, while a related conversation happened, the translation to the parent was not wholly accurate. It is not uncommon for a child to "tell" on the parent or to believe that the therapist can "make" or persuade the parent to give them what they want. The therapist cannot be an arbiter between the parent and child, although they can facilitate conversations. Clear communication, with delineated limits, can help with this issue.

Whose Therapist Am I? How Do I Deal with Conflicts When They Arise?

The line between being the child's therapist, with conjoint parent guidance, and being the parent's therapist can get blurry if you are taking on both roles. Be continually mindful of the work that you are doing with each member of the family. There are times when the work with the caregiver involves addressing their own mental health needs in service of helping the child. Unlike with individual psychotherapy, there is a potential for conflict when this situation arises.

STRATEGY: *Keep Your Eye on the Child Patient*

Keep the focus on the child whether you are doing stand-alone parent guidance or parent guidance as an adjunct to child therapy. Talk with the family about the work you are doing, and explain that should the need arise you will refer them to their own therapist even if you maintain your parent guidance role. Other reasons for a parent therapy referral may include: when the parent's needs are so great that they overshadow the other work you are trying to do; when the struggles, needs, and what is best for the parent are in conflict with those of the child; or when one party repeatedly shares secret information about the other.

Watch for a dynamic in which the child or caregiver is using your therapy to achieve goals that are different from those that you have agreed on. Sometimes child patients tell their parents that we actually endorse something that we may only have empathized with, to get something else they hoped for. For example, they may suggest that we recommend a mental health break from school, a pet, or dying hair. In this situation, it is an advantage to have ongoing contact with the parent and child so that you can clarify your role as a supporter and not a parental decision maker. Sometimes parents also wish for us to "get their children to do something" or for us to find out and report back on their children's secrets. Both scenarios can be sticky. Talk with the parent and child about your need to maintain a strong therapeutic alliance with all parties, which would be undermined by being the lieutenant or spy for the parent or a decision-maker.

Cultural and Demographic Differences in Parenting

JDS was given a baby sling as a gift before the birth of her first child. When she visited a family friend, who is a Western-trained pediatrician, and carried her child in the sling, she was asked, "Won't the baby fall out?" The answer is no. When she attended a community organization meeting, wearing the baby in the sling, a group of Ghanaian mothers approached her and showed her additional ways to use the sling. They had never spoken with her before, but this parenting behavior became an important point of connection. Though the baby sling made the Western-trained pediatrician nervous, it made the Ghanaian mothers comfortable.

Learning about different cultural values and beliefs can assist in planning parenting interventions. For example, a therapist was encouraging a family to help their child, a gifted musician, to perform more solos and seek more "starring" roles in his youth orchestra. The family did not follow up on these recommendations. When the therapist queried the parents, they explained that they preferred that their child learn to be a part of the group, rather than seek to be the one gaining the most attention. The parents, who were Japanese American, explained their differing philosophy. They encapsulated the different beliefs by comparing two sayings: the Japanese concept that "the nail that sticks up gets pounded down" in contrast with the American saying that "the squeaky wheel gets the grease."

Religious beliefs may also come into play. If you have little knowledge of particular beliefs, or struggle to determine how they can be incorporated into treatment, if they need to be, it can be worthwhile seeking consultation from a knowledgeable source such as a religious leader. We are working within a value-laden sociocultural context. Parent guidance, similar to all psychotherapy, is subject to cultural bias. The histories of our professions, the histories of different populations, and our own subjective lens all influence the work we do.

Match or Mismatch?

When parents seek guidance, they are not only looking for a skilled therapist, they also are looking for someone who will understand their experience. We cannot always match our clients in terms of demographics or experience with a particular concern. Letting families know that we have some basic understanding is important. While it can feel empowering and validating for a clinician to listen to and learn from families, the experience can also be burdensome to the clients. For example, if you are working with a family of color and you do not have a basic awareness of relevant topics, including current events, historical issues, and microaggressions, you may do this family a disservice.

A parent may seek out a clinician who matches them with regard to demographics or identities, so that they can feel assured that the clinician understands their experience from the start. There are many issues faced by parents who are not of the dominant race, who do not have privileged backgrounds, who belong to different ethnic groups, or have different gender identities. They have to do with experiences that they have had, doors that have not always been open to them, and messages that they have been given about who they are and how they should behave. Not understanding those concerns can create significant problems, including a rift in the therapeutic relationship or a mismatch between the interventions and the needs of the clients. Since we know that parenting is an area that differs across cultures and subgroups and is already rife with the opportunity for judgment, be careful not to reinforce those experiences or messages. The results of the 2015 Report of the U.S. Transgender Survey note the high number of respondents who had negative experiences in a health care setting in the previous year (James et al., 2016). As therapists, we do not want our work to add to someone's bad experiences.

Given that it is unlikely that we match our clients on all relevant demographic characteristics, we should be mindful of how to handle mismatches. Neither of us has matched all of our clients with regard to age, ethnicity, religion, racial identity, gender identity, or sexual orientation. How do you send the message that diversity is welcome in your space? How do you indicate that you are interested in learning what you do not know about their personal experiences without putting an undue burden on the client? Intersectionality takes into account the multiple aspects of people's identities that combine to influence their experience of discrimination and privilege (Crenshaw, 1989). Their experience is created through the interplay of varied factors.

STRATEGY: *Create a Welcoming Environment*

Think about creating a welcoming place for your diverse clientele, including representation in your physical space. What kind of artwork, other decorations, and reading material do you have in your office? What books do you have? What words do you use when you connect with parents before you actively begin the work?

STRATEGY: *Educate Yourself*

If a parent is coming into your office with an experience that you know nothing about, educate yourself. Between what can be learned from colleagues and the internet, information is typically easily accessible. Do not create a burden for your clients to educate you.

When clients feel misunderstood or invalidated, acknowledge these feelings. Many people appreciate our candor about what we don't know. When you, as the clinician, bring difference into the room, it gives permission for the clients to talk about it more comfortably. It lets them know that you recognize these dynamics. Talking about it demonstrates your understanding of the impact of difference, as well as your commitment to using that understanding to inform the work you will do together. Sometimes, individuals may not want to work with a therapist who lives in their own community because the community they come from is small. Do not assume what people will want. Check in with them.

Be cautious about chalking up unexpected behavior or attitudes to the family's cultural background. Community members, including mental health professionals and clergy, can help a clinician clarify these concerns. Of course, information about a client should not be shared with someone in the community. Instead, you can use skillful internet searching or ask experts nonidentifying questions to help determine whether a behavior, cognition, or reaction is within expectable norms for their group.

There are values and beliefs about how children should be raised that vary across cultures and subcultures. Ask yourself whether these values are just different from what we are used to or whether they are antithetical to how we work. If they are just different, then you may need to adjust how you typically work to be culturally responsive. However, if they are antithetical to how you work, then talk with the family and discern whether it makes sense for you to work together. For example, many parents have reported that their parents used spanking as a punishment, without a negative outcome. Without being judgmental, you can say something like "In clinical practice, we have not found spanking useful, as it can have a negative impact on your relationship and does not tend to be very effective. I'd like to work with you on other forms of discipline." If you can offer other interventions that increase their control, they may have a much easier time giving it up.

Environmental, Economic, and Structural Limitations

Outside stressors add to the challenges of our work. Families with more financial resources can devote more time to the work you are asking them to do. They may also be able to purchase rewards for a system you create and hire advocates or add out-of-pocket services, such as occupational therapy and executive-functioning coaching. Families with more limited resources may not be able to afford additional help, which will require you to be creative. What outings in your area can you suggest that a family can do for free? Does a museum offer free admissions one day per month in the summer? Does the family's insurance company offer case management or other wraparound services that would aid the family and make your work more feasible?

In our experience, there are some communities that have more fear of agencies than others. They may have more experiences with child protective services in their circle. They may have concerns about their legal status.

STRATEGY: *Be Aware*

Target your interventions to the resources that the family can employ. Be sensitive to worries about social service agencies, politics, and policies. Be aware of the policies where you work regarding whether law enforcement has the right to come to your office and ask for clients' records. Let the parents know about policies with respect to confidentiality. You can, then, allay fears to the best of your ability.

WORKSHEET 17.1

In My Parent Guidance Work I Am Struggling with . . .

- I don't feel like treatment is progressing.
  - ◆ I am feeling this way because . . .
  - ◆ I can . . .
  - ◆ What would help is . . .

- I feel like this person puts up a brick wall to every suggestion I make.
  - ◆ I am feeling this was because . . .
  - ◆ I can . . .
  - ◆ What would help is . . .

- I feel angry or distressed when they tell me about how they handled a situation.
  - ◆ I am feeling this way because . . .
  - ◆ I can . . .
  - ◆ What would help is . . .

- I feel frustrated by their lack of insight.
  - ◆ I am feeling this way because . . .
  - ◆ I can . . .
  - ◆ What would help is . . .

- I feel like this parent does not respect me as a skilled therapist.
  - ◆ I am feeling this way because . . .
  - ◆ I can . . .
  - ◆ What would help is . . .

- I feel like it is hard to set clear boundaries with this parent.
  - ◆ I am feeling this way because . . .
  - ◆ I can . . .
  - ◆ What would help is . . .

WORKSHEET 17.2

Parent Guidance Pitfalls Check-In

Pitfall List

- therapist as expert
- therapist as judge
- the wayward therapist
- runaway train
- dialectics of parenting
- no "therapeutic contract"
- roles and conflicts
- Wile E. Coyote
- control freak
- mismatch
- family calls you out on a mistake
- therapist as better parent than parent
- therapist as friend
- Johnny One-Note
- problematic reactions
- parents have trouble agreeing
- COW
- the stonewall
- the wet noodle
- the martyr
- situational stress
- legal and ethical concerns

I see a pitfall ahead!

Which one? ____

How do I avoid it? ____

____

I am in a pitfall!

Which one? ____

How do I get out of it? ____

____

I was in a pitfall!

Which one? ____

What did I learn from it? ____

____

CHAPTER 18

Legal and Ethical Concerns
Avoiding Dangers and Reducing Risk

Doing parent guidance requires consideration of dual relationships, boundaries, roles, and confidentiality: the legal and ethical aspects of this work. Each clinical discipline has its own code of ethics. Become familiar with the principles laid out in the relevant codes as well as federal and state laws and regulations.

What You Should Consider from the Codes of Ethics

The National Association of Social Workers (NASW), American Psychological Association (APA), American Mental Health Counselors Association (AMHCA), American Association for Marriage and Family Therapy (AAMFT), and American Counseling Association (ACA) all have codes of ethics that share a number of common concerns (National Association of Social Workers, 2017; American Psychological Association, 2017; American Mental Health Counselors Association, 2020; American Association for Marriage and Family Therapy, 2001; American Counseling Association, 2014). While these ethical concepts are relevant to all psychotherapy, there are specific concerns related to parent guidance work.

Informed Consent

All professional codes of ethics discuss informed consent. Obtaining informed consent is critical in managing the issues of risks and ethics. Pay attention to the word *informed*. As the therapist, you may have a clear expectation moving forward, including both what you will do and what the family will do. However, this process may be very new to them. Use the informed-consent process to develop expectations, including clarifying roles and relationships, and to discuss privacy, confidentiality, and the limits of confidentiality. Keeping in mind the dynamic nature of the work we do, continue to update informed consent when you revisit goals, roles, expectations, and other relevant aspects of treatment. The informed-consent process involves anticipating questions and concerns.

STRATEGY: *Informed Consent as an Ongoing Process*

Treat informed consent as an ongoing process, not a static one, that begins immediately. You can think of informed consent as a beneficial part of the treatment, given that it helps to explain the parent guidance process and set expectations. Review the information in your documentation, such as treatment and fee agreement, confidentiality, your role and the family's role in treatment, what the family can expect, how parent guidance works, and setting goals. Setting up and managing expectations provide a foundation that both you and the family can refer back to. Revisit these issues as circumstances change and evolve, bringing up changes with families as they occur so that they can ask questions, clarify information, and share concerns. When parents are adequately informed, they have the opportunity to ask questions that help them engage more fully in the treatment. Center the "informed" aspect of informed consent. The following case study provides an example of informed consent in practice.

CASE STUDY: Who's the Client?

A clinician was working with a child in therapy. To enhance the effectiveness of the therapy, the clinician engaged in some additional parent guidance work with the mother. Before adding the parent guidance work, the therapist spoke with the mother about the two roles: as child therapist and as parent coach. The therapist also discussed the advantages of seeing a different provider for parent help and the risks in doing parent coaching as an adjunct to child therapy. After having a few sessions of parent guidance to work on parenting without the child present, the mother shared information regarding intense negative feelings about the child and did not want the therapist to bring that information into therapy with the child. The mother was also beginning to reveal issues from her own childhood, which did impact her parenting but required more work in individual therapy. The therapist said to the mother, "We had talked about the times when it would not make sense for us to do this work together. Some of those things have come up now." The therapist further explained, "I am glad we were able to talk about your child, as it helped clarify that you still have feelings about your own childhood. You may benefit from working on these issues with your own therapist. As we discussed at the start, since my focus is on helping your child, I will refer you to a colleague so you can have the attention to your needs as you deserve." Although the mother was disappointed because she felt very comfortable with the therapist, the possibility that she would be referred to individual therapy had been stated at the outset as part of the informed-consent process. The mother was not surprised and accepted the referral. When she started her own therapy, the parent guidance therapist agreed to communicate with the new provider in order to help this transition happen smoothly.

Confidentiality and Access to Records

Confidentiality

Therapists need to be straightforward about confidentiality and the limits thereof with all family members at the outset. When doing parent coaching, the clinician will need to clarify, in their own mind, as well as for the family, what information will be shared clinically and how it will be shared. For example, when a parent tells you something about the child's behavior without the child present, how will you handle this disclosure? Or perhaps the child tells you something that the parents did which runs counter to what you had agreed they would try, and the parent does not share this information with you. Use your informed-consent process to explain your policies for sharing information, talking through how you intend to handle information in a legal, ethical, and therapeutic way. Clarify not only the legal aspects of confidentiality, but also, in practice, how you handle burdensome information. Burdensome information, in this case, is information that one family member shares with the therapist that is being kept from other family members. While discussing confidentiality is always important, when multiple members of a family are involved, there are more opportunities for different family members to "confide" in the therapist. This may result in the therapist having information that is difficult to deal with in the context of working with the other family members, and opportunities for missteps in sharing information may be greater than encountered when doing individual work.

Consider this example: A mother calls the therapist to tell her that her child, the identified patient, has not been turning in homework and has been lying to the mother and the therapist for weeks. Schoolwork and homework had been the focus of treatment, and the child had been telling the therapist that they were on top of things, that everything was going well, and that they are feeling good about school and communicating with their family. The mother reveals that the child is not following through as they had promised. How does the therapist handle this information?

Ideally the therapist has talked ahead of time with the child and the mother about how the sharing of information will be handled. In this moment, the therapist asks the mother if the child knows that she is sharing this information. If the mother says yes, this admission makes it easy for the therapist to bring it up with the child. A conversation could start with something such as "So, you know your mother called me. Let's talk about what she told me and see what we want to do with this information." If the mother says no, the therapist would explain to the mother that, unless the child can know that the therapist has been told, it is hard to do anything useful with the information. The therapist can talk to the mother about how to bring the child into the conversation. The child also needs to know that information will not be communicated through secret channels.

Another example occurred when JDS was part of an outpatient adolescent DBT team. An adolescent presented to this DBT program because of self-injurious behavior, using cutting regularly as a means to self-soothe and regulate. As part of the routine treatment in a DBT program, JDS asked the adolescent to complete daily diary cards on which they logged whether they engaged in self-injurious behavior. She then used the diary cards in session. As a parent, JDS knew that the adolescent's parent might want to know every time a cutting episode happened. As a therapist, she knew that when doing parent guidance, if she reported every cutting episode to the parent, the adolescent would not let her know about this behavior very often.

It was necessary to have an explicit conversation involving the adolescent, the therapist, and the parent at the start of the treatment about what JDS would share with the parents, what she would not share, as well as the reasons for her decision. She explicitly stated that she would not tell the parent every time the adolescent let her know that they cut, as doing so would interfere with treatment success. She let them both know the circumstances under which she might handle the matter differently, such as if the adolescent needed medical attention or if concern about suicidality shifted significantly. They came to an agreement, and then, despite what the parent might have preferred, they understand the reasons for why sharing information about the behavior was handled this way were clear. JDS also documented the conversation.

Always address concerns, such as parents wanting to know about behaviors that their child discloses to you. You can give them an example, such as "A parent might ask me 'Is my child dating *X* again?' and I would say 'As we discussed, your child has to feel comfortable talking with me and knowing that I won't share what we talk about unless it falls into a category of things I would share. It's hard not knowing details of your child's life that you are worried about. Let's figure out how to talk to your child about that."

Access to Records

There are federal and state regulations regarding access to records. Discuss how information sharing will be handled, not only with regard to records, but also regarding information that you will share with collateral contacts, such as medical personnel and school staff.

Exchanging information with collateral contacts helps with improving your formulation and planning interventions. A family may have given you a release of information to talk with the child's school staff or some other collateral party. Even if the release is written for "the entire record" be cautious about sharing only information pertinent to that individual and for the purpose of the conversation. It becomes easy to partner with collateral contacts and, in doing so, essentially gossip about a family. Sometimes in an effort to increase a collateral contact's empathy for a family situation, we may be tempted to share more information than is necessary and therefore appropriate. This kind of partnering can have harmful outcomes. For example, sharing a parent's trauma history may inspire more sympathetic attributions but is not directly related to the child and would likely lead the parent to feel exposed. Instead, saying something such as "the parent has their own history that may be influencing their response. Let's figure out the best way to move forward to help this family" may be more helpful. The parent has likely shared more about themselves with you, as a parent guidance therapist, than they have with other adults in their child's life. That is important for our work, as well as a privilege and an honor that we must respect.

When the parent has significant mental health concerns, it is even more important to be clear about what information to share with collateral contacts. For example, does the school staff need to know about the sexual abuse history or diagnostic history of the caregiver? EB once worked with a father who had his own significant mental health issues, including paranoia. She had worked hard to develop a strong relationship with him and was successful enough that he signed a release for her to talk to his child's school staff. At one point, she had a conversation with the school team who, in turn, talked to the father and, in their efforts to compel different parental behavior, misquoted what she told them. This breach served to undermine EB's relationship with the family, and she had some repair work to do to regain their trust.

STRATEGY: *Confidentiality*

When a child is involved in therapy, the therapist is acutely aware of the access that the parent or guardian has to the record. When the child turns 18, they will have access to their own record. If you have been providing parent coaching in the child's name and documenting those sessions in the child's record, the child may have the opportunity at some point to see your documentation. Keep in mind who will have access to your written record as you document your parent coaching sessions.

Multiple Relationships

When working with children and consulting with their caregivers, think through what relationships you will have with each of the family members. According to Standard 3.05 of the APA Code (APA, 2017, p. 6), "A psychologist refrains from entering into a multiple relationship if the multiple relationship could reasonably be expected to impair the psychologist's objectivity, competence, or effectiveness in performing their functions as a psychologist, or otherwise risks exploitation or harm to the person with whom the professional relationship exists." Other disciplines' codes of ethics have similar language. In parent guidance work, clarify the roles and relationships with the multiple parties involved. Be clear regarding whose therapist you are. You may be the child's therapist, offering guidance to the parent(s), the parent's therapist working on parenting among other things, or another therapist working specifically on parenting. Keep in mind the "reasonable expectation" language. A conceivable pitfall here is the potential for conflicts of interest and lack of clarity on the part of the family members, which could lead to confusion and upset.

It can be problematic to hold multiple roles. For example, it may be worth stating that, should it become apparent that the parent would benefit from individual therapy, you will refer them to another therapist. If you are considering doing both the child's individual therapy and the parent coaching, think about whether you can be the best therapist for the child and the best parent guidance clinician at the same time, when there may be conflicting needs and desires.

In contrast, sometimes serving in both roles can give you a unique vantage point, allowing you to be more successful with both the parent and the child. Take a child who presents with anxiety and also identifies as gender nonbinary. In an attempt to be helpful and supportive, their parents made an appointment at a gender clinic that treats children and adolescents medically for gender dysphoria. The child told the therapist that they did not feel the need for any medical interventions, identifying as gender nonbinary and being happy with their body. This was helpful information that the therapist was able to, with permission, talk through with the parents during parent guidance sessions.

CASE STUDY: A Therapist of One's Own

A trainee was seeing a child for therapy because of oppositional behavior at home with his mother. The trainee worked with the child to better understand the reasons for his anger outbursts and to help him develop more positive coping skills. As part of this treatment, the trainee engaged the parent in monthly sessions to discuss the progress in the child's therapy and to improve the parent's support for the child's change efforts. This mother, though loving toward her child, struggled with mood regulation. She became very dysregulated, both with the child and the trainee therapist, during therapy. In the first meeting, the mother yelled at and insulted the trainee. Over time, the trainee developed an understanding of the mother's struggles and considered providing her with individual therapy. The therapist thought that difficult interactions with this mother were inevitable, and given that they had already gone beyond those initial interactions they could move more quickly toward productive psychotherapy. She was tempted to shift from parent guidance to individual therapy because she saw the mother's difficulty in connecting with professionals and also the significant progress she had made in parent guidance.

However, in consultation with her supervisor, the trainee realized that she could not support both the mother and the child. She determined, with her supervisor's help, that a conflict of interest was foreseeable, as it was likely that the child and the parent would have conflicting needs at times, placing the therapist in a bind and likely rendering both of the therapies ineffective. The trainee continued with parent guidance and referred the parent to a colleague in the same clinic, sitting in on the first session in order to help the mother feel comfortable and engaged. A year later the mother acknowledged that it was meaningful to have her "own" support person, whose primary focus was on her and not on behavioral improvement for her child.

STRATEGY: *Be Clear and Communicate*

Both for yourself and with the family members, be clear about and communicate what your role will be with the family members. In our training, we learn about roles, conflicts, and multiple relationships. Our clients do not. Educate them about these issues so that they better understand the decisions and recommendations you are making. If you foresee your role shifting, explain that as well. Try to ensure that your clients understand your role and the goals in the work you are doing.

EB worked with an adolescent to address his OCD symptoms and provided weekly parent guidance work to reinforce exposure practice. The teenager resolved most of the symptoms, completing his therapy. The discussion turned to termination. The mother excitedly stated, "Now that he's no longer anxious and doesn't need therapy anymore, can we be friends?!" In this situation, EB had to address the roles and issues here. While the adolescent was the identified client and the parent guidance work was ancillary to the child therapy, a professional and clinical relationship still existed. How the therapist conceptualized her role vis-à-vis the mother was different from how the mother thought about it or hoped it could be. Simply because the mother is not the identified patient does not mean that we do not consider that we have a professional relationship meriting the same considerations as the relationship with the identified patient. The therapist had to explain to the mother that the boundaries still existed.

While typically therapists work with only one member of a family, some therapists manage the role of "the family therapist," similar to the family doctor, not in the sense that they are doing family therapy, but in the sense that they are serving as the therapist for multiple family members. It is especially important when engaging in such an endeavor, to be thoughtful about roles and boundaries. A situation in which one might work with more than one member of a family could come about when the therapeutic alliance with one family member enhances the alliance with another and there are no foreseeable conflicts of interest. Therapist availability may also factor into this decision making.

When thinking about your role, it can help to ask yourself these questions:

- Whose therapist am I?
- Does meeting with the child help their mental health and behavioral functioning?
- Would adding in parent guidance boost the efficacy of the child's treatment?
- Would it be more effective to meet with just the parent?
- Is parent guidance turning into individual therapy for the parent?
- Are the child's needs and parent's needs at odds?
- How do I feel about this parent and child?
- Am I able to maintain professional boundaries with the parent (i.e., not too casual)? If not, why?
- If I am asked to do, or feel inclined to do, something that I do not typically do (such as buy a gift, attend an event), would doing something atypical be in my patient's interest or my own?

Managing risk requires the ability to think through the ethical and legal issues of our fields and manage them in the best ways possible. Parent guidance, because it involves multiple family members, may make issues around confidentiality, roles, goals, and relationships more complicated. Use the informed-consent process to establish clarity around roles with all appropriate family members. It is common for parents to wish to "have more" of you as an individual therapist. When this issue arises, remember to consult when you are unsure and to document your decision-making process, including with whom you consulted, what decision you made and why, and what you decided not to do and why. Use Figure 18.1 to assist in being intentional about decisions surrounding risk management.

- "Have I done a thorough informed consent?"
- "Have I talked through confidentiality with all family members in developmentally appropriate ways?"
- "Have I explained mandated reporting?"
- "What is my role with and my relationship to each family member?"
- "Does everyone understand my role?"
- "If I shift roles, do the family members understand and agree?"
- "Have I clarified all legal issues, including custody issues?"
- "Am I clear on who is involved in parenting?"
- "Have I worked to involve everyone who should be involved, even if it is challenging?"
- "Have I documented discussions and decisions, including both why I did what I did and why I did not do what I did not do?"

FIGURE 18.1. Watching my own back in parent guidance: Questions for risk-management self-check.

PART VII
PACT in Action

Throughout treatment keep the question of "how will we know when we are done?" in mind. In this part, we discuss evaluating when to stay the course and when to end treatment. We also provide a case example using PACT and explicate the decision-making process throughout the case.

CHAPTER 19

Assessing Progress and Ending Treatment

Evaluating Progress: Staying or Changing the Course

PACT: "T" for "Treat and Terminate"

Therapists should continuously assess whether parent guidance is working to meet the goals set in early sessions. Elicit feedback, both informal and, if appropriate, formal, throughout the therapeutic process and use the feedback to inform your coaching. This is an iterative process, with adjustments being made at any point in the process, as indicated by data along the way. The assumption that you just get to the end of treatment and, in a perfunctory way, do an outcome measure to tell you what you already know (that things are better), is overly simplified and not particularly useful.

If the expected change is not occurring, consider the possible barriers. Why is the family struggling to implement the intervention? The why will guide you to the next steps. There may be practical barriers. If there are, determine whether they can be solved. If barriers cannot be removed and remain a problem, consider whether another intervention will better fit the family situation. For example, when recommending more child-led play between caregiver and child, sometimes parents just cannot get themselves to take the time to do it. If they cannot, and you have done troubleshooting that addresses both the emotional and practical barriers with the parent, recommend something else. In one family the parent did not engage in child-led play, citing a lack of time. Instead, the clinician recommended taking the child on errands to the grocery store. The parent and child both loved it. It was not precisely the same recommendation, but it was an intervention that actually happened!

There are many reasons that an intervention does not work. It is possible that the family does not understand the recommendation, which leads to ineffective implementation. Probe for details about what they are doing. We have frequently heard parents say that they have tried everything. Perhaps, for example, the therapist recommended that the child do their homework at the kitchen table so that the parent is more available if the child needs help. The specifics of how they implemented the recommendation can be enlightening. When you inquire further, you learn that the parent is on their phone when the child is doing homework, and they happen to also be working with the child on not interrupting. Hence, the parent is not actually available to the child during homework.

The family is likely doing the best they can. Treat each case as a single-subject research study. You start with the evidence-based techniques but if they are not leading to the results you want, you can adjust and try something else. Troubleshoot by returning to the basics. Ask yourself these questions about the lack of effective progress in parent guidance:

- **P:** Do you have a successful **p**artnership with the parent? Do they come to appointments ready to work? Do they ask questions and have ideas? Do they try agreed-upon suggestions? If they do not, why not? Does the parent appear engaged? Do they forget appointments?
- **A:** Do you feel you have accurately **a**ssessed and understand what is going on with the parent and their child? Do you have enough information? Has your formulation of the problem changed? Do you and the caregiver have a shared vision of the difficulties?
- **C:** Did you make a clear **c**hoice of how to intervene? Was your choice informed by your partnership and assessment of the presenting problem? Do you have the parent's buy-in?
- **T:** How did the execution of your chosen **t**reatment work? Did the parent consistently follow through with the intervention strategy? Did you accurately assess barriers? How did you evaluate the success of the intervention?

Measuring the Effectiveness of the Intervention: How Do Parents and Clinicians Know If the Interventions Are Creating Positive Change?

Data obtained directly from the family provides informative feedback that can be used to determine whether to stay the course or try another intervention. The process of eliciting feedback from the family is both informative and continues to let them know that their opinion is critical. You can obtain feedback formally, such as through client satisfaction surveys or pre- and postmeasures, or informally throughout the process.

The feedback that you elicit should relate to the achievement of goals and objectives. At the start of parent guidance, you create a treatment plan with goals and objectives that spell out where you are going with your work. It is good practice to regularly review them with the caregivers in order to make sure that you continue to agree on what you are doing. Together you can reflect back and consider whether the goals and objectives have been met or if they need to be revised over time. Concluding together that the goals have been met will be the determining factor regarding whether treatment is complete, whether less frequent maintenance treatment is warranted, or whether new goals can now be the focus of treatment. When your review of progress, goals, and interventions reveals that the intervention is not proceeding as desired, identify where the problem may lie, and reenter any of these stages of the treatment process. You can then "choose" again based on your assessment of what went wrong.

Measurable goals make it easier to assess progress. Gathering baseline data will help as well. For example, when doing your assessment, if the parent expresses concern about tantrums, ask how frequently they happen, how intense they are, how long they last, and how long it takes the child to recover. These are all measures you can refer back to during treatment. You may discover that although a caregiver tells you that the intensity and duration of the tantrums have remained the same, the frequency has dropped from about once per day to once per week. The parent may also say that the frequency of tantrums remains the same but the intensity and duration are reduced, making the tantrums less exhausting for all. Both of those outcomes represent marked improvement!

The measures of improvement in Figure 19.1 were developed with the help of many participating parents in a group therapy program that ran over multiple years.

1. There is less anger at home.
2. There are fewer reactions that are disproportionate to the triggers.
3. Transitions work better.
4. There is more flexibility in the family.
5. The child is better able to express their feelings.
6. The child shows greater confidence.
7. The child is able to solve problems.
8. The child successfully previews activities.
9. There is more family frustration tolerance.
10. The family uses more positive language and less derogatory language.
11. The child is motivated to learn and make things work more smoothly at home and school.
12. Activities of daily living (dressing, brushing teeth, getting up in the morning, going to bed at night) go more smoothly.
13. There is less stress for family members.
14. Everyone is happier.
15. There are quiet times at home.
16. The child makes fewer negative comments about themself and more positive remarks about themself.
17. Evening times go more smoothly.
18. Siblings have good times together.
19. The child is more easily redirected.
20. The child is more aware of their feelings/behavior in the moment.

(continued)

FIGURE 19.1. Some measures of improvement in parent guidance.

21. There are fewer outright tantrums, they have less "volume" (defined as less aggression, less destruction, and lasting a shorter amount of time), and there is a quicker recovery to baseline.
22. Parents feel less isolated.
23. Parents feel in control of home life.
24. Parents feel that they have a strategy that works.
25. Parents have time to take care of themselves.
26. Family members are able to invite friends over.
27. The child feels comfortable outside of the home.
28. Family members take responsibility for their actions.
29. Family members take each other's perspectives.
30. Parents look forward to spending time with the child.
31. Parents have less guilt about their parenting style.

FIGURE 19.1. *(continued)*

When you use parent-guidance outcome measures, think about who is reporting and what information they are providing. Some measures are global measures of functioning or well-being. Others focus on specific signs, symptoms, and diagnoses. If you have measures from multiple reporters, do they correlate with each other, or do they seem to be talking about different children? If they seem to be talking about different children, that fact may tell you something about environmental impacts on behavior, requiring more assessment and a new formulation. If, however, the measures are consistent with each other, then that is helpful in terms of formulation, as well as with regard to evaluating progress. Additionally, outcome measures can facilitate a conversation with the parent and/or the child about how you are seeing what is happening and how they are seeing the situation.

CASE STUDY: Improvement: Expected and Unexpected

A mother seeks psychotherapeutic help for herself and her 7-year-old daughter, who has significant anxiety and clinginess. This behavior is impacting their morning routine, as the child is afraid to go to school, starting the day on a difficult note that continues until nighttime, making even bedtime challenging. Using an outcome measure (such as the Revised Children's Manifest Anxiety Scale—Second Edition [RCMAS-2]; Gurley, 2011), you gain a baseline rating of the child's anxiety. This measure shows that the biggest issue is separation anxiety, which aligns with the rest of the information obtained in the evaluation. After establishing rapport with the family, assessing, and developing your formulation, you establish the goals. You strategize with the mother about helping the child go to school with less stress and anxiety and about developing a consistent bedtime routine. After setting goals, treatment begins. In order to achieve the goals, the parent guidance includes coaching the mother on how to develop and use routines, preview with the child, manage parent affect around her child's anxiety, manage the anxious moments with the child and use exposure and shaping to reduce her child's anxiety around school and bedtime. In sessions with the mother, feedback suggests that the child is going to school more easily and going to sleep independently. The mother is very proud of her daughter, who is, in turn, proud of herself. You readminister the RCMAS-2 and find that the child falls below the clinically significant threshold on all of the anxiety scales. Finally, the mother reveals that she and her daughter both enjoy the pleasant evening routine. It feels relaxed, especially now that they have more time in their day, given the reduction in tantrums and anxiety. The treatment is complete.

In this example, the positive time spent between the mother and her daughter, though not a direct target of intervention, improved dramatically. Even when you are not focusing on the caregiver and child relationship, consider these interactions as part of your assessment of outcome, as it is likely that when other problem areas improve, the amount of enjoyable time between the parent and child will also improve.

Effective Termination

The goal of parent guidance is to improve the situation such that you are no longer needed and the parent functions well on their own. Keep in mind the question "how will we know when we are done?" Do not surprise the caregiver with a happy statement of "Well, I was looking at your treatment plan and you seem to have met all of your goals, so today is our last session. Hooray!" This is a collaborative endeavor from start to finish.

We might suggest using the word *transition,* rather than *termination.* The word *terminate* has a finality that can be off-putting to caregivers. Challenging as it may be to strike the perfect note for each parent, we can think about some ways to handle ending an episode of parent guidance treatment that may be more effective.

Think about the ending of parent guidance as an important, and not just perfunctory, part of the therapeutic process. Sometimes we mark the end of a treatment episode with an activity or ritual, an item they can take with them, such as a polished stone, or simply a review of the work and the significance of the change that has occurred. Be thoughtful about how to mark this transition. Do not set it up as a forever good-bye. Sometimes new issues appear, and parents need a "booster." There may be the one-time return to work on a new issue or on the resurgence of an old symptom. You might also have a parent who comes in periodically for bursts of treatment as different issues arise in their lives. You want them to feel welcome to come back if they feel the need to.

Returning to parallel process, think of a transition out of an episode of treatment as akin to launching, as we hope parents might launch a child. This transition does not mean that the child can never come home again, but it does means that they have mastered the necessary skills to be more independent in a significant way, an occasion worthy of marking. Similarly, the parent has reached a level of competence to succeed on their own. They can do something else with their time, other than spend it in parent guidance.

EB was consulted by a parent who had done effective and positive work with another therapist. The son had separation anxiety that was impacting the whole family. They worked well with the therapist, who did both individual work with the child and coached the parent on how to support the child. The treatment progressed, everyone was very happy with the result, and the treatment ended. Later another issue cropped up with this parent and child, but the family was not comfortable returning to the previous therapist. The problem was, thinking that a reward would be wonderful, the therapist created a big "graduation" ceremony for him and his parent. It was such a big deal that the family was too embarrassed to return to the former therapist, concerned that a return would let him down. Clearly, this was not the therapist's intent, but there was an unforeseen consequence of what seemed like a positive ritual.

Termination can be difficult for the therapist. It can be sad saying good-bye to parents whose lives we have impacted and who, in turn, have impacted us. We may have encountered a family with whom we worked very well. We may be proud of both the parents and the child, how far they have come, and how much happier they are. Still, it is time for them to launch. Termination may also be difficult for the client. In the context of parent coaching, the caregiver may feel that they are losing a partner. They had a confidante who did not judge their parenting, someone who gave them genuine feedback and assisted them in making improvements without making them feel like they were going it alone. Having someone who hears them without being judgmental may be unique for the caregiver. It is not unlikely that other people, including friends, family, and perhaps strangers, have judged their parenting behaviors. These positive feelings may be lost when the therapeutic relationship comes to a close. Think about how they can hold onto you, as an appropriate attachment figure, when they are no longer working with you. Set up that transition well, so that the client feels successful and ready to go, but also so that they know that the door can be open to them if needed.

Additionally, consider what the parents will be losing, both in terms of the specific therapeutic relationship and also with regard to other, ancillary gains. Some parents develop lovely rituals around appointments that may disappear if they are not intentionally continued. Both authors know families who enjoyed the time in the car together before and after appointments and would get food either before or after sessions. Continuing these therapy-related traditions is important, despite no longer coming to scheduled appointments.

A clinician had provided parent guidance and individual therapy for a boy with ADHD. The treatment included consultation with the parents regarding managing his activity level, building organizational skills for schoolwork using planners, adding family routines around mealtimes and homework, bringing him onboard to increase his motivation around relationships and his future, and teaching him skills to delay gratification. The treatment was deemed successful and it ended. Years later the parents called the clinician and asked to be seen. The original identified patient was a young adult and had died suddenly of a previously undiscovered genetic condition. After he died, other members of the family were discovered to have the condition as well. The parents requested help with their grief, as well as with managing the anxiety about the other affected family members. They felt that, because this clinician knew the family and the young adult who had died, they wanted to be seen by that same clinician. This new episode of treatment was short term and focused.

Parent guidance is not typically a forever endeavor, and termination may not be either. JDS once received a phone call from a mother she had worked with a number of years earlier. The mother had had a significant medical event and wanted to tell the clinician. She voiced, "You know everything else about us. I felt like you should know this too." A strong connection had remained for her. A supportive conversation ensued. She was not seeking any additional treatment, just that connection. Both the treatment and the termination years before had been successful, and the mother did not need more than to share this news. The whole process, from partnering and assessment to treatment and transition, holds a very important place for the caregivers with whom we work.

CHAPTER 20

Using PACT to Steer Your Integrative Parent Guidance

A Case Example

The Framework for Intervention

- Partner
- Assess and formulate
- Choose the intervention
- Treat and evaluate outcomes

Partnering is the recognition of the critical relationships involved in helping children and their parents via parent guidance. Changes occur in the context of a trusting relationship between a provider and caregiver.

Understanding the problem and its context in detail is essential for developing and choosing an optimal treatment plan. With a knowledge of current parenting techniques, attachment styles, and child and parent mental health, you can perform a detailed assessment and formulate a strategy that identifies the ways the parent can shift what they are doing to improve the situation for everyone.

The partnering and assessment stages form the groundwork for choosing the best path for intervention. Using your expertise and your formulation, you thoughtfully develop a plan to recommend to the caregiver.

Once you have chosen an intervention, you can begin treatment. As you deliver parent guidance, consider whether the treatment is creating the desired outcome. A regular accounting of the progress being made is critical for guiding the intervention on the most efficient and positive path.

Although the PACT framework is not typically articulated in our work, we believe that PACT is the ideal way to conduct parent guidance. We believe that the critical components we suggest make parent guidance work more successful. These components include knowing where to begin (partnering with parents), knowing what you need to know (how to assess), knowing how to put it together (formulate), knowing what to do (choosing the intervention), knowing how to move forward (intervene), and knowing when you have accomplished what you set out to do (measuring success).

Note that the steps of PACT build on one another. You do not stop partnering with parents once you start the assessment, and your assessment may deepen as you get to know them. You intentionally choose and apply the intervention for treatment, measuring whether your approach is effective or needs to be adapted. Consider these tasks as discrete but intertwined, beginning sequentially but continuing simultaneously.

Decision Tree for Parent Guidance Interventions

Once you have decided that parent guidance is an appropriate intervention, there are questions you can ask yourself to make certain you are heading in a positive direction:

- Is there a clear presenting parent guidance problem? If so, are there barriers that will inhibit treatment?
  - If there are barriers, address them first.
- If there is not a clear presenting problem, are there multiple issues, or is it not apparent what they need help with?
  - If there are multiple issues, work with the parents to prioritize and then treat them.
- If the issues are not clear, think about whether you need to do an extended formal assessment phase or whether there is something you can start treating, as you continue to get to know the parents.
- If there are no barriers to treatment, or you have addressed the barriers, then consider intervention options.
  - Would this presenting problem benefit from:
    - Improving parenting through the teaching and building of skills?
    - Addressing it as a usual suspect?
    - Trying a behavioral intervention?
    - Is there a widely accepted best practice for this presenting problem?
  - If so, are you skilled at using the technique(s) best suited for the problem? If not, can you learn them, or be supervised adequately to use them?
  - When you decide on a treatment path, talk with the family about the approach you would like to take and, if they agree, treat.
  - If you are not skilled in the appropriate area or able to learn the needed skills, refer the family to another clinician and talk to them about your reasons for doing so.
- Do you need to choose among multiple treatments? If so, consider the strengths of and the demands of each one, and which one will fit best with your formulation. Choose the treatment and talk to the caregivers about the approach.

Integrative Parent Guidance Using PACT: Case Example

Keeping PACT and the decision tree in mind, we consider a case example. The parents of 6-year-old Aisha sought help to manage her oppositional behaviors. Aisha was diagnosed at birth with numerous congenital anomalies, and additional medical issues that required medical procedures arose in her preschool years. She was noncompliant and aggressive with her parents, the hospital staff, and her teachers.

Would Integrative Parent Guidance Help?

Although Aisha was young, she was able to engage in some level of individual psychotherapy. In an initial evaluation session, she was oppositional with the therapist, refusing to answer questions but she would engage in play. When her parents joined in the session to try to increase her comfort, she calmed briefly, but seemed to have very little ability to process her feelings. When asked directly if she wished to have fewer tantrums, she ignored the question. The therapist then introduced play, which calmed Aisha, and her play themes included traumatic medical interventions. The therapist believed that a trauma-informed or play-based approach might in the future provide some therapeutic benefit for Aisha.

Aisha's parents discussed the urgency of their need for help. The medical team was becoming increasingly frustrated with her inability to tolerate medical procedures without restraint. Aisha's parents, in contrast, were very motivated to help her feel less distressed and to improve their own situation by reducing her oppositionality at home. It was noteworthy that they described significant discord between themselves. In this situation, it was very likely that a key intervention to improve Aisha's behavior would be parent guidance. Let us look at how PACT was used in working with this family.

Partner

The family was struggling. The clinician, Nicholas, met them, listened to their story, and conveyed his understanding of the difficulties with Aisha. He instilled hope through his commitment to hearing their story in depth and by developing a concrete plan of action to assist them in intervening with her going forward. Nicholas took notes as they spoke, clearly respecting their detailed knowledge of their daughter's development. He commented on the challenges in raising a child with such significant medical needs, which her parents had prioritized to keep Aisha as healthy as possible. Nicholas was patient in his initial session with the parents, not moving to a more formal assessment stage until he recognized the partnership with and comfort level of both parents.

Assess and Formulate

After gathering assessment information and hearing the parents' story about raising Aisha, Nicholas began to ask his own questions about the parents, Aisha, and the running of the household. Aisha was an only child with no known cognitive or learning challenges. Using the standard assessment questions, Nicholas discovered that there was significant stress and conflict between the parents, who had little family support, as neither of them felt close to their own parents. Each parent was also raised in a household where their own parents had fought, divorcing when each of Aisha's parents were children. They described their own upbringings as strict but with little involvement from their parents when they were growing up. Aisha's father reported that he felt that he was learning to parent from books and the internet because he did not want to repeat the patterns that were modeled by his own parents. Aisha's mother, with a lower-paying job, bore the brunt of handling Aisha's medical treatments and appointments. The conflict between the parents was palpable, even during the assessment, as they disagreed about how to manage Aisha, which they noted led to yelling and name calling.

The mother had a strong drive to correct earlier mistakes. She felt tremendous guilt because she had gotten angry with Aisha when she was younger for moving slowly and complaining about stomachaches. Years later these symptoms were connected to medical diagnoses. Aisha experienced medical trauma during her many procedures, which included the use of multiple restraints. Her parents felt helpless in improving her ability to cope with these feelings. Continued medical procedures were unavoidable because Aisha's medical problems were serious. Aisha and her family needed help to refine parenting skills, to improve Aisha's behavior, to help her cope with future procedures, and to assist in processing her trauma.

Choose

Given the family presentation, the urgent need for progress around the family dynamics, and Aisha's medical adherence, parent guidance was a necessary adjunct to Aisha's individual psychotherapy. Aisha participated in individual sessions, at the start, to address her medical trauma. After thinking about the primary presenting problems (oppositional behavior, parent conflict and inconsistent responses to Aisha, medical trauma, and anxiety about ongoing medical care), Nicholas spoke to the parents about his recommendations, including parent guidance. The work involved the following elements to address the presenting problems:

- *Improving parenting skills, including improving collaboration and reducing conflict.* Nicholas discussed the benefits of having a clear and explicit parenting plan, which would be a start toward reducing conflict. He discussed some typical parenting skills that would benefit the family. There was no routine around bedtime, which was one of Aisha's "usual suspect" difficulties. The parents were eager to come to an agreement about the best ways to manage nighttime, including taking turns about who would read a story to Aisha, which previously had not been a consistent part of the routine. In addition, they set a regular bedtime with Nicholas's help, which increased the amount of sleep Aisha was getting each night and allowed the parents time to be together.

However, the tension between the parents not only involved raising Aisha. As a result, Nicholas also referred the parents to a colleague for couples therapy.

- *Processing parent feelings.* Aisha's parents had mood regulation issues with regard to handling Aisha's behavior and illness. The feelings underlying these issues had been, for the large part, unspoken. Her father did not realize that his wife was struggling with guilt about her earlier management of Aisha's behavior. Indeed, Aisha's mother was not consciously aware of how preoccupied she was with guilt. She was also surprised during this early choosing phase of treatment that her husband did not know how she felt. They both felt disrespected by Aisha's behavior toward them and embarrassed about her behavior toward other people.

- *Parent management of Aisha's behavior at home.* Aisha's parents had inconsistent responses to her difficult behavior at home. Sometimes they appeased her by giving her whatever she wanted in order to stop her tantrumming and name calling in the short term. They tried ignoring her, though she often then engaged in dangerous behaviors that were unsafe to ignore. At other times, they yelled, took away screen time and favorite toys, and told her how bad her behavior was in an attempt to shame her into better behavior. Neither parent had a clear plan to manage her negative behavior or to build positive behavior at home.

- *Parent response to Aisha's medical trauma and ongoing medical needs.* Nicholas spoke with Aisha's medical providers to gain an understanding of what her current medical needs were as well as to understand what she would face in the near future. Given her medical illness, Aisha would require monthly blood work and follow-up appointments as well as more invasive procedures at times. This knowledge informed his decision to recommend trauma work.

Treat and Measure Outcomes

Nicholas talked to the parents about these different foci for treatment. The parents agreed with all of the interventions suggested by Nicholas. They included Aisha in the conversation about what her therapy would focus on and also let her know that Nicholas would be meeting with them as well in order to help them be more helpful for Aisha's behavior. Recognizing that there were several important goals, they prioritized them together and got to work.

- *Improving parenting skills, including building collaboration rather than conflict within the family.* Nicholas worked with the parents on implementing child-led play in order to improve overall family interactions. The parents started couples therapy, and as their relationship began to improve, they also became more open to shifting some of the patterns at home. The bedtime routine was going better as they reported to Nicholas in a session. When Aisha had more sleep, it appeared to help in other areas of her functioning as well. In addition, the nighttime reading as well as child-led play were beneficial in Aisha's relationship with both of her parents. The parents were also choosing videos to watch together after Aisha went to bed, which improved their relationship. Nicholas encouraged the parents to stick with these new family patterns.

• *Processing parent feelings.* Although both parents still had some negative feelings about Aisha's behavior and the onset of her medical illness, they became more aware of these feelings. Aisha's father, with his newfound awareness of his wife's stress, offered to take Aisha for her next blood draw. Nicholas suggested to the parents that Aisha's behavior at home was more problematic because she was closer to them than to other adults, and not because she wanted to be disrespectful. With this new attribution, the parents appeared to feel less distressed by her behavior toward them. Nicholas reviewed the interactions over the week with the parents. He worked with Aisha's mother to shift her thoughts and feelings, via cognitive restructuring, He helped her recognize that she had not been intentionally mean but rather, did not understand the nature or severity of Aisha's medical condition.

• *Parent management of Aisha's behavior at home.* Nicholas talked about the benefits of a consistent and positive response to Aisha's challenging behavior, and the parents agreed to try to "catch her when she's good." Nicholas also provided education on behavioral reinforcement systems, which he planned to implement in the early stages of the treatment.

With the strategy of "catch her when she's good," both parents noticed more times when Aisha was actually behaving well and following the family rules. After a few weeks of improving Aisha's sleep, the parents decided to embark on a more structured reinforcement plan. With Nicholas's help the parents identified one behavior (going to her cozy corner and reading when upset) to reinforce and drew a sticker chart with Aisha. The chart allowed her to earn three stickers a day for going to the cozy corner and reading instead of hitting. If she did not get upset at all at the end of the day she could put an additional three stickers on her chart, a requirement that they felt was important because they did not want Aisha to appear upset just so she had the opportunity to earn stickers. Aisha responded well to booming praise, which the parents provided, along with a sticker every time she stopped tantrumming and went to the cozy corner. After she received 12 stickers, Aisha and her parents would go to a movie. Aisha's parents reported that she was very proud when she showed the sticker chart to her grandparents. The parents also scripted their response to negative behavior when it did occur in this part of the treatment phase: "You'll have another chance to go to the cozy corner later today if you would like."

• *Individual therapy and family consultation around Aisha's medical trauma.* With Nicholas's help in her own individual therapy, Aisha revealed her worries concerning her medical procedures. Nicholas used an evidence-based model to address Aisha's medical trauma. She enjoyed developing her trauma narrative and looking forward to how her story might help other children who have to endure many similar procedures. Her fears subsided, and her compliance improved. Nicholas and Aisha involved her parents in this work, so that they better understood her behavioral responses and how to support her. They also explained Aisha's fears to her medical providers, who demonstrated a more empathic stance when they understood how she felt.

The parent guidance work with Nicholas helped the parents to recognize and manage their own affect so that the home environment was calmer, which modeled more effective affect management for Aisha. Her parents were also able to better attend to her needs when their own emotions were managed more effectively. The overt conflict in the home was reduced. Once they seemed to solve the bedtime problem, Nicholas helped them develop new routines for typical days as well as for the ongoing medical procedures. They talked through what to do when unpredictable events occurred.

With regard to measuring outcomes, Nicholas and the family were concerned with reducing Aisha's oppositional behavior and increasing comfort with medical procedures. When reviewing the progress on these goals each week with Nicholas, the parents defined what measures of progress they could use as benchmarks: how many weekly tantrums Aisha had and how many times she needed restraints during blood draws. They also talked about the benefits of other referrals, such as the couples counseling and individual therapy for the mother if she wanted to further process her parenting guilt. The parents saw an improvement in family interactions; a reduction in Aisha's oppositional behaviors at home and school and in the hospital setting; more positive behavior and play with parents; and improved adherence to medical procedures. Life still had challenges for them, but parent guidance made a big difference. Aisha and her parents completed treatment, having made significant progress.

In Conclusion

Parenting in Unusual Times

As we wrote this book, we were in the midst of unprecedented political times, climate concerns, and a global pandemic. All of these factors have impacted parent guidance work. Parents look to us as experts to advise them about how to manage their own feelings and talk to their children about these world events. This can be challenging as we too likely have strong feelings, which we need to manage those during sessions. The pandemic has changed how we do this work, and it has also put additional strains on mental health professionals trying to meet the needs of so many who are struggling. The caregivers with whom we work may have handled COVID-19 safety differently from the way you did or in a way you thought was unwise. When we provide parent guidance, we need to recognize the realities of a particular situation: We may have previously worked very hard with a family to limit screen time for academic and social reasons, but the pandemic may have upended that intervention plan.

Regardless of what unusual circumstances exist in the times we live, they will impact treatment. We need to understand the realities of what parents are dealing with and take them into account when planning our interventions.

Mary Poppins as Parent Coach

If you have not seen the film *Mary Poppins,* it is worth viewing from a professional perspective. When the seemingly magical nanny first joins the Banks family, the parents are indulgent, neglectful, and judgmental. During Mary Poppins's time with the family, the children experience a structured and warm caregiver, and their obedience improves. The parents also learn a different parenting style. Despite the fact that the family will miss her terribly, in the end she leaves, because she is no longer needed. As in the film, the critical relationship between the parent and child remains when the therapist is no longer a part of the picture. The therapist, like Mary Poppins, may be missed, but this work was never really about the therapist. Ultimately, the therapist leaves the family with the skills to function well and happily together. Just as Mary Poppins left the Banks family once she had provided all that they needed, we end this book hoping that you have acquired additional skills to enhance your professional practice.

APPENDIX A

Resources for Clinicians

Books to Assist with Parent Guidance

Blaustein, M., & Kinniburgh, K. M. (2010). *Treating traumatic stress in children and adolescents: How to foster resilience through attachment, self-regulation, and competency* (2nd ed.). Guilford Press.

Blaustein and Kinniburgh describe their approach, ARC, for helping traumatized children. Their approach includes caregiver guidance as a significant piece of the intervention strategy, and they offer many tools toward that end.

Cohen, J. A., Mannarino, A. P., & Deblinger, E. (Eds.). (2012). *Trauma-focused CBT for children and adolescents: Treatment applications.* Guilford Press.

Cohen and colleagues teach trauma-focused CBT (TF-CBT) by demonstrating the applications of their model in helping traumatized children.

Creswell, C., Parkinson, M., Thirwall, K., & Willetts, L. (2017). *Parent-led CBT for child anxiety: Helping parents help their kids.* Guilford Press.

Creswell and colleagues describe the step-by-step use of cognitive-behavioral therapy (CBT) by parents to help their anxious children.

Faber, A., & Mazlish, E. (2012). *How to talk so kids will listen & listen so kids will talk.* Scribner.

Faber and Mazlish's classic parenting book teaches optimal communication skills for parents to use with their children in an engaging cartoon format.

Ginott, H. (2003). *Between parent and child: Revised and updated: The bestselling classic that revolutionized parent–child communication.* Three Rivers Press.

Ginott's timeless text, originally published in 1965, has helped parents learn to speak empathically to their children for over half a century.

Gray, C. (2015). *The new social story book, revised and expanded 15th anniversary edition: Over 150 social stories that teach everyday social skills to children and adults with autism and their peers.* Future Horizons.

This book provides social stories and instruction about how to use them to help young children and those with autism spectrum disorders navigate a variety of situations.

Greene, R. W. (2016). *Raising human beings: Creating a collaborative partnership with your child.* Scribner.

Greene, the developer of Collaborative Problem Solving/Collaborative and Proactive Solutions, describes his approach to building positive parent–child relationships.

Huebner, D., & Matthews, B. (2005). *What to do when you worry too much: A kid's guide to overcoming anxiety.* Magination Press.

Huebner and Matthews have created a series of "what to do when" books, often utilizing CBT techniques, that parents can use to help children tackle common child concerns.

Kabat-Zinn, J., & Kabat-Zinn, M. (1998). *Everyday blessings: The inner work of mindful parenting.* Hachette.

This book applies mindfulness to parenting. Jon Kabat-Zinn also has books and audio programs to assist adults with mindfulness.

Linehan, M. (2015). *The DBT skills training manual* (2nd ed.). Guilford Press.

Linehan, the originator of dialectal behavior therapy (DBT), presents resources, worksheets, and handouts that can be reproduced and used with parents to understand and implement DBT.

March, J. S., & Benton, C. M. (2007). *Talking back to OCD: The program that helps kids and teens say "no way"—and parents say "way to go."* Guilford Press.

March and Benton provide a well-tried approach to reducing symptoms of OCD in children and teenagers.

McNeil, C. B., & Hembree-Kigin, T. L. (2010). *Parent–child interaction therapy* (2nd ed.). Springer.

Early proponents of PCIT describe the approach in depth.

Rapee, R., Wignall, A., Spence, S. H., Cobham, V., & Lyneham, H. (2009). *Helping your anxious child: A step-by-step guide for parents.* New Harbinger.

This book is written for parents to help address their child's anxieties with a systematic approach.

Whittingham, K., & Coyne, L. W. (2019). *Acceptance and commitment therapy: The clinician's guide for supporting parents.* Academic Press.

Whittingham and Coyne teach acceptance and commitment therapy (ACT) to clinicians who wish to use this approach as part of parent guidance.

Games to Recommend to Families

- *Charades* is a game that involves paying attention to the other players. Both the person acting out the clues and the audience need to attend closely to other people and think about what the other person may be thinking.
- *Snail's Pace Race* (for three to six players) is a game that minimizes the focus on winning. While not a cooperative game, it can be played in multiple ways. In one version, the goal of the game is to guess which snail will cross the finish line first. In another version, a

different goal is that the last snail to cross the finish line wins, so the object of the game is to be last.

- Cooperative board games. When playing cooperative games, all players win or lose as a team. Players help other players and can make suggestions to each other. Because of the cooperative style of game play, often children younger than the recommended ages can play these games. Three examples of cooperative games are:
  - *Castle Panic* (one to six players)
  - *Forbidden Island* (two to four players)
  - *Pandemic* (two to four players)

Websites to Help Parents and Clinicians

Common Sense Media

This website provides a wealth of information for clinicians and parents with regard to media for children and teens. It reviews all media (movies, books, television shows, apps, and podcasts) and provides a synopsis of the content. It has a "What Parents Need to Know" section for every review, noting the age the material would be appropriate for. It also indicates positive and beneficial messages in the media.

Do2learn.com

Do2learn advertises itself as a "resource for individuals with special needs." The site has games, activities, and resources for building social skills and developing emotion recognition, helping with behavior management, and other issues. It can be used by clinicians, teachers, and families.

Gamer Dad

"Andrew Bub" has been providing information and advice about video games since 2003. His website offers information about the pros and cons of games as well as their appropriateness for different age groups. He enjoys the games and at the same time presents a valuable perspective on content that may not be appropriate.

Reachchild.org

This Canadian website, created by child development specialists, offers a great deal of material to help find apps, websites, social stories, and home activities for children. It pays special attention to resources for children with developmental and mental health concerns.

Relaxation Resources for Parents and Clinicians

This is not an exhaustive list of available relaxation, meditation, and mindfulness resources. There are many books, YouTube videos, podcasts, and apps to assist clinicians in teaching parents and children these important skills. These are a few that we have found helpful.

Calm

Calm has a free trial option but then charges a fee for ongoing use of all of its resources. With audio and video programs geared to improving sleep, mental health, and overall functioning, it is a favorite for many clients. Teens are attracted to some of the celebrity (Shawn Mendes) mindfulness meditations.

Headspace

Headspace is a tried-and-true website/app that also has a free trial option and then charges a fee for ongoing use. It has mindfulness and meditation programs for different amounts of time that can help improve mental health.

Lori Lite's Stress Free Kids

Lori Lite has created books and audio programs to assist younger kids in learning relaxation, in using positive affirmations, and in reducing stress. The CDs (Indigo Dreams and Ocean Dreams) can also be downloaded on iTunes.

Ten Percent Happier

More than 500 meditations, including some for sleep. The website and app have a free trial, with additional fees for meditations, podcasts, and courses.

Review Article

Weekly, T., Walker, N., Beck, J., Akers, S., & Weaver, M. (2018). A review of apps for calming, relaxation, and mindfulness interventions for pediatric palliative care patients. *Children, 5*(2), 16.

This article provides a review of many online programs for relaxation that can be useful for both a medical population and healthy children.

APPENDIX B

Other Services a Family May Benefit From

There are many other services that a family may avail themselves of in order to help their child. We include descriptions of these services and the reasons for referring families to them.

Group Services

When you believe that a parent or a child would benefit from talking with others in similar circumstances, or you find that they are very isolated and feel alone in dealing with their issues, consider referring them to a support group or clinical treatment group. Groups may be a useful adjunct to the work you are doing. In reviewing the literature, Worrall et. al. (2018) find that a range of support groups are effective in many ways, including for fostering hope, building strategies, and improving mental health. Support groups exist for most illness groups, mental illness categories, learning differences, behavioral challenges such as addiction and life circumstances, LGBTQ identities, and grief. The focus of support groups varies: Some include sharing resources, some offer clinical suggestions, or some involve creating a community that has experienced a similar circumstance. Though the quality varies, caregivers may profit from talking with others in similar situations who can communicate their shared experiences. Some therapeutic groups may be centered around teaching a particular skill set, such as a parenting technique like collaborative problem solving, or a method of intervention, such as dialectical behavior therapy (DBT).

Medication Evaluation

When you believe that a parent or child has significant issues that would benefit from a medication approach, consider referring them for a psychiatric medication evaluation. Consider a psychiatric medication referral for children or their parents when there is acute suffering that may improve more quickly with medication, if the use of medication will allow the client to better access psychotherapy or reduce the risk of a dangerous behavior, and when there is evidence that the symptoms in question (such as attentional difficulties and anxiety) are very likely to be improved with medication. When there are mild symptoms that may respond to behavioral interventions alone, you may suggest that children and their parents try psychotherapy for a period of time before considering medication. However, there are times when therapy is not progressing as expected, and we recommend a medication evaluation sooner. However, making a referral for a psychiatric medication evaluation only means that you are suggesting the family to obtain information, rather than actually recommending that they consider a specific medication. Parents may have strong feelings about medication—interpreting it as a failure in parenting, as a sign of a lifelong disability, or as "poisoning" their child with a dangerous substance—which you can help them understand and manage. It can be important to let them know that an evaluation is not a commitment to trying medication.

Medication is usually not the first choice of parents who are seeking psychotherapy because of its risks and side effects. Medication can help alleviate symptoms, but it does not replace psychotherapy. Rather it can help the parent and child make better use of therapy. Take, for example, the child whose anxiety is so debilitating that they are not able to use the techniques that you have taught the parents to facilitate. The parents are expending energy managing day-to-day life with their child. Medication may reduce the anxiety enough that the child is able to practice the techniques, such as exposure to mildly frightening situations, that will ultimately pave the road to recovery. Further, the parents can shift their approach from comforting the child, fighting figurative fires or managing frequent disruptive behavior or panic, and avoiding feared situations to actively cuing the child to use the techniques discussed in sessions.

Medical Specialty Evaluation

When you believe that a parent's or a child's difficulty is medically based, consider a referral for a medical evaluation. Issues can present in ways that seem to be mental health concerns but are actually medical in origin. There are times when you need to consider whether there may be a medical concern, given how the parent or child presents. In general, a change in functioning around toileting, eating, sleeping, energy level, or mood would benefit from ruling out any medical reason that these changes may have occurred, especially when there does not seem to be any environmental trigger. Surprisingly, these evaluations may not be seen as important, although they can be central to why a person is not currently doing well emotionally. For example, thyroid conditions can affect energy, mood, and sleep (Capetillo-Ventura & Baeza, 2014). Bed-wetting and behavior changes can be early signs of diabetes (Kahanovitz et al., 2017). Neurological conditions are often accompanied by a change in behavior. In general, a sudden behavior change may have a medical underpinning that is often worthwhile to have checked by a physician. Know what the local specialty clinics can offer. Consider these specialized evaluations:

- *Audiologists.* Not hearing well can impact a number of areas of functioning. We often see a difficulty with language development in children as one manifestation of a hearing difficulty. Behavioral outbursts, because of difficulties with communicating, are also seen in some young children who are not hearing well. In addition, children with central-auditory-processing disorders also show difficulties in school and at home. Audiologists can assess these areas.

• *Ophthalmologists.* Sometimes vision issues can cause headaches and emotional difficulties for adults and children. Squinting may be a cue. Surprisingly, people are not always aware that they are not seeing well.

• *Dietitians (nutritionists).* Poor nutrition can be a sign of a depressive mood or an eating disorder, but it can also cause mood dysregulation. A dietitian can help in making a food or eating plan when children are not getting the proper nutrition. Psychotherapists can then help a child and the family implement the recommendations made by a dietitian. Parents are critical in implementing nutrition recommendations for their children.

• *Sleep experts.* Similar to the impact of poor nutrition, inadequate sleep has an effect on mood and behavior. Although many sleep problems have to do with ineffective bedtime routines when standard interventions are not working, it may be time to consider a medical evaluation focused on sleep. Though the interventions of a sleep expert may be similar to those of a therapist, they can also look at any potential neurological factors. They also have access to sleep studies that can determine some of the biological contributions to the child's sleep difficulties.

• *Pain treatment specialists.* At many major hospitals, there are pain treatment programs to help manage the psychological factors involved with chronic pain. In these interdisciplinary programs, a team of professionals works to understand the response to pain and endeavors to increase effective functioning since chronic pain often removes people from their everyday environments. Chronic pain has a clear impact on mood and behavior (Pascali et al., 2019).

Other Specialized Evaluations

When you believe that further evaluation would help you more effectively choose interventions, consider a referral for a specialized evaluation. Sometimes a significant role for the therapist is identifying evaluations that would lead to a more complete formulation and that can help define the next steps for the parent and child. When you are meeting with the caregiver, consider what information would be useful for them and their child. Consider these specialized evaluations:

• *Psychological and neuropsychological assessments.* Psychological testing can be a helpful adjunct to parent guidance when it would be useful to get a measure of the child's or parent's cognitive abilities and how that measure interfaces with personality, coping, daily functioning, and other areas of concern. If you suspect ADHD, executive functioning issues, memory problems, a nonverbal learning disorder, or a brain-based contribution to difficulties or need more information about how cognition and personality are affecting the person, testing can be very valuable.

Critical to knowing what kind of testing to refer someone to is knowing what questions you want answered. There are several types of psychological testing that are available to patients, including psychological testing, neuropsychological testing, educational testing, and developmental testing. Psychological testing often includes basic cognitive or intelligence testing, as well as tests that look at personality style, current preoccupations, how people perceive and understand the world, and coping styles. Neuropsychological testing also includes intelligence testing, but it adds a much more complete assessment of cognitive strengths and weaknesses, including executive functioning, learning and memory, visuospatial skills, language skills, and approach to tasks. Educational assessments can be part of either psychological or neuropsychological testing or can be performed on their own. These tests more specifically aim to evaluate the child's academic or educational attainment, which are helpful when you are uncertain about the child's match with their school and/or grade level.

• *Speech and language evaluations.* If there are concerns about speech or language development, then an evaluation by a speech and language pathologist would be appropriate. Speech and language pathologists can assess a number of areas, including speech production, receptive and expressive language, and social pragmatics (the social use of language). When children cannot communicate their wants and needs, there may be a speech or language problem, not an issue with respecting parents, managing behavior, or something else targeted in psychotherapy. Speech and language concerns are relevant to behavioral functioning, because difficulty understanding or expressing oneself verbally can lead to problematic behavior, sometimes without an apparent antecedent. Speech and language pathologists also provide evaluations and interventions in the areas of social pragmatics and executive functioning (discussed further below). If you are concerned about the child's ability to understand (receptive language), or express themselves (expressive language), or their capacity to use language skillfully for social interactions, then this kind of evaluation is an important adjunct to parent guidance.

• *Occupational therapy.* Occupational therapists (OTs) evaluate fine motor skills, sensory concerns, and activities of daily living skills. OTs can work with children on improving fine motor and movement skills. If you find that children are hypersensitive to sounds, sensations, colors, clothing tags, or foods, it may be worthwhile to obtain a referral for an OT evaluation. It can also help improve parent and teacher empathy by understanding that children's reactions are based on their processing of sensations, rather than interpreting them as attempts to annoy others.

• *Physical therapy.* Physical therapists (PTs) examine gross motor skills. Often physical therapy may be provided after an injury to promote recovery or for people with delayed gross motor skills or physical disabilities, such as cerebral palsy. Your advocacy of and knowledge about these services can help families navigate them.

• *Executive functioning.* Executive functioning (EF) is a relatively new field of evaluation and intervention. Parents and children may be identified as having EF difficulties in the areas of self-management, goal setting, taking initiative, staying focused, managing emotions, seeing the bigger picture, and managing frustration (Dawson & Guare, 2018). These difficulties are most often identified when people are less successful than expected based on their cognitive profile. EF coaches, who are sometimes psychological professionals or speech and language specialists, focus on "how" things are done rather than on the content of what is done. An EF coach can help organize work content or space, set priorities of what task to tackle first, or help the child to be aware of how much time each task takes. Although psychotherapy can help a child in setting priorities, it is generally not as focused on improving work or academic success in this way.

• *Social pragmatics.* There is a burgeoning field of social thinking and social pragmatics, popularized by speech and language therapist Michelle Garcia Winner (2007). If you discover that your patients do not have friends or appear dumbfounded by regular interactions, consider an evaluation of social pragmatics. Social pragmatics focuses on the functional use of language in connection between people. People who have difficulties in this area may have trouble expressing themselves and making friends, and appear unusual, because their behavior may be "unexpected," which is Winner's word to describe behavior in less judgmental ways. Social therapy evaluations, group therapy, or social coaching can be very beneficial when people have trouble figuring out what to say, following the rules of communication such as conversational turn taking, and using language to maintain relationships. As in working with EF deficits, a therapist may introduce some of these skills, but when a lack of social interaction skills is the predominant issue, it is often better to refer to a coach or group with a specific focus in this area.

Educational Services

When the child and family need help with school-related issues, consider referring them to the following services.

- *School-based evaluations and interventions.* Be aware that parents can access for free many of the evaluations and interventions that we have described in public schools. Schools can provide OT, PT, speech and language therapy, educational remediation, and help with social and emotional concerns. In providing parent guidance, you should be aware of the Individuals with Disabilities Education Act (IDEA), which ensures that students are entitled to "FAPE" (a free and appropriate education) to meet their needs. Schools in different districts and states may have their own process for developing individualized education plans (IEPs). Know the laws and processes where you practice.

- *Educational advocacy.* Since we are neither educational advocates nor attorneys, we will often refer to or partner with these professionals to help caregivers access the best educational plan for their child. Educational advocates are trained to understand relevant laws and regulations regarding education and special education in order to navigate the special education process. They can also coach parents to be better able to advocate for their child in the school system. As the parent guidance expert, you are likely not as familiar with the intricacies of the school system and the regulations.

- *Attorneys.* When consulting an advocate does not yield the result of an appropriate educational placement or plan, attorneys may be helpful in promoting school compliance with relevant regulations. Sometimes caregivers engage attorneys around issues related to severe bullying, interacting with the child welfare system, or housing disputes. Lawyers can also assist when clients are either victims of crimes or accused of misbehavior that has legal ramifications. In general, when there is an issue that would benefit from legal advice or engagement, referring to a lawyer is helpful. Many areas have free or low-cost legal aid services.

Other Programs a Family May Ask About

When you are asked about what additional programs are available, you should know about the following types of programs.

• *Experiential, adventure-based programs.* There are other programs that families may ask for your opinion about, including experiential, adventure-based programs like Outward Bound; meditation, music, or other expressive therapies; and equine (horse) therapy. When thinking about these alternative programs, consider whether there are data to support their efficacy. It may be beneficial to speak with a program representative directly to learn about it and assess whether it makes sense as an adjunctive treatment.

Sometimes parents choose interventions for the family or child that can actually be harmful. For example, professional organizations have made statements about programs such as "conversion therapy," wherein the goal of the program is to change someone's sexual orientation. The American Psychological Association (2009) "concludes that there is insufficient evidence to support the use of psychological interventions to change sexual orientation." When interventions seek to erase a person's identity without their consent, be very wary.

You can use Worksheet App.1 to help you consider referral services for clients.

WORKSHEET APP. B.1

Clinician Worksheet: Potential Other Referrals for This Family

Concern	Recommended service	Family interest	Disposition

References

Acri, M. C., & Hoagwood, K. E. (2015). Addressing parental mental health within interventions for children: A review. *Research on Social Work Practice, 25*, 578–586.

Ainsworth, M. D. (1963). The development of infant–mother interaction among the Ganda. In B. M. Foss (Ed.), *Determinants of infant behavior* (pp. 67–112). Wiley.

Ainsworth, M. D. S., Blehar, M. C., Waters, E., & Wall, S. (1978). *Patterns of attachment: A psychological study of the strange situation*. Erlbaum.

Aktar, E., & Bögels, S. M. (2017). Exposure to parents' negative emotions as a developmental pathway to the family aggregation of depression and anxiety in the first year of life. *Clinical Child and Family Psychology Review, 20*(4), 369–390.

Alvarez, E. T., Muñoz, M. Z., Moraga, M. J., & Garcia Alvarez, J. (2015). The effectiveness of relaxation techniques in anxiety disorders. *European Psychiatry, 30*, 1112.

American Academy of Child and Adolescent Psychiatry. (2020). Screen time and children. Retrieved February 11, 2023, from *www.aacap.org/AACAP/Families_and_Youth/Facts_for_Families/FFF-Guide/Children-And-Watching-TV-054.aspx.*

American Academy of Pediatrics. (2021). Family media plan. Retrieved February 11, 2023, from *https://www.healthychildren.org/English/fmp/Pages/MediaPlan.aspx.*

American Association for Marriage and Family Therapy. (2001, July 1). AAMFT code of ethics. Retrieved February 11, 2023, from *www.aamft.org/resources/lrm_plan/ethics/ethicscode2001.asp.*

American Counseling Association. (2014). 2014 ACA code of ethics. Retrieved February 11, 2023, from *www.counseling.org/knowledge-center.*

American Mental Health Counselors Association. (2020). AMHCA Code of Ethics, Revised 2015, 2020. Retrieved February 11, 2023, from *www.amhca.org/viewdocument/2020-amhca-code-of-ethics.*

American Psychological Association. (2009). Insufficient evidence that sexual orientation change efforts work, says APA. Available at *www.apa.org/news/press/releases/2009/08/therapeutic.*

American Psychological Association. (2017). Ethical principles of psychologists and code of conduct: Including 2010 and 2016 Amendments. Retrieved February 11, 2023, from *www.apa.org/ethics/code.*

Anton, C., & Lewis, S. (2017). *A smart girl's guide: Digital world; How to connect, share, play and keep yourself safe*. American Girl.

Bar, S., Milanaik, R., & Adesman, A. (2016). Long-term neurodevelopmental benefits of breastfeeding. *Current Opinion in Pediatrics, 28*(4), 559–566.

Barkley, R. (2013). *Defiant children: A clinician's manual for assessment and parent training* (3rd ed.). Guilford Press.

Barr, R. G., & Fujiwara, T. (2011). Crying in infants. In C. D. Rudolph, A. M. Rudolph, G. E. Lister, L. R. First, & A. A. Gershon (Eds.), *Rudolph's pediatrics* (22nd ed., pp. 318–321). McGraw-Hill.

Baumrind, D. (1971). Current patterns of parental authority. *Developmental Psychology, 4*(1, Pt. 2), 1–103.

Beck, J. S. (2020). *Cognitive behavior therapy* (3rd ed.). Guilford Press.

Biglan, A., Flay, B. R., Embry, D. D., & Sandler, I. N. (2012). The critical role of nurturing environments for promoting human well-being. *The American Psychologist, 67*(4), 257–271.

Blaustein, M. E., & Kinniburgh, K. M. (2010). *Treating traumatic stress in children and adolescents: How to foster resilience through attachment, self-regulation, and competency*. Guilford Press.

Bowlby, J. (1988). *A secure base: Parent–child attachment and healthy human development*. Basic Books.

Bowling, A., Slavet, J., Miller, D. P., Haneuse, S., Beardslee, W., & Davison, K. (2017). Cybercycling effects on classroom behavior in children with behavioral health disorders: An RCT. *Pediatrics, 139*, e20161985.

Brandon, A. R., Pitts, S., Denton, W. H., Stringer, C. A., & Evans, H. M. (2009). A history of the theory of prenatal attachment. *Journal of Prenatal & Perinatal Psychology & Health, 23*(4), 201–222.

Buist, K. L., & Vermande, M. (2014). Sibling relationship patterns and their associations with child competence and problem behavior. *Journal of Family Psychology, 28*(4), 529–537.

Cataudella, S., Lampis, J., Busonera, A., Marino, L., & Zavattini, G. C. (2016). From parental–fetal attachment to a parent–infant relationship: A systematic review about prenatal protective and risk factors. *Life Span and Disability, 19*(2), 185–219.

Chess, S., & Thomas, A. (1984). *Origins and evolution of behavior disorders: From infancy to early adult life*. Harvard University Press.

Choate, L. H. (2016). *Swimming upstream: Parenting girls for resilience in a toxic culture*. Oxford University Press.

Chua, A. (2011). *Battle hymn of the tiger mother*. Penguin.

Cole, P. M., Dennis, T. A., Smith-Simon, K. E., & Cohen, L. H. (2009). Preschoolers' emotion regulation strategy understanding: Relations with emotion socialization and child self-regulation. *Social Development, 18*(2), 324–352.

Compernolle, S., DeSmet, A., Poppe, L., Crombez, G., De Bourdeaudhuij, I., Cardon, G., . . . Van Dyck, D. (2019). Effectiveness of interventions using self-monitoring to reduce sedentary behavior in adults: A systematic review and meta-analysis. *International Journal of Behavioral Nutrition and Physical Activity, 16*(1), 63.

Crenshaw, K. (1989). Demarginalizing the intersection of race and sex: A black feminist critique of antidiscrimination doctrine, feminist theory and antiracist politics. *University of Chicago Legal Forum, 1989*(1), 139–167.

Dawson, P., & Guare, R. (2018). *Executive skills in children and adolescents: A practical guide to assessment and intervention* (3rd ed.). Guilford Press.

De Shazer, S., Dolan, Y., Korman, H., Trepper, T., McCollum, E., & Berg, I. (2021). *More than miracles: The state of the art of solution-focused brief therapy*. Routledge.

De Varis, J. (1994). The dynamics of power in psychotherapy. *Psychotherapy: Theory, Research, Practice, Training, 31*(4), 588–593.

Dearing, E. (2004). The developmental implications of restrictive and supportive parenting across neighborhoods and ethnicities: Exceptions are the rule. *Journal of Applied Developmental Psychology, 25*(5), 555–575.

Denham, S., Workman, E., Cole, P., Weissbrod, C., Kendziora, K., & Zahn-Waxler, C. (2000). Prediction of externalizing behavior problems from early to middle childhood: The role of parental socialization and emotion expression. *Development and Psychopathology, 12*(1), 23–45.

Domingues-Montanari, S. (2017). Clinical and psychological effects of excessive screen time on children. *Journal of Paediatrics and Child Health, 53*, 333–338.

Doran, G. T. (1981). There's a S.M.A.R.T. way to write managements' goals and objectives. *Management Review, 70*, 35–36.

Dweck, C. S. (2008). *Mindset: The new psychology of success*. Ballantine Books.

Eyberg S. M., & Bussing, R. (2011). Parent–child interaction therapy for preschool children with conduct problems. In R. C. Murrihy, A. D. Kidman, & T. H. Ollendick (Eds.), *Clinical handbook of assessing and treating conduct problems in youth* (pp. 139–162). Springer.

Faber, A., & Mazlish, E. (2012). *How to talk so kids will listen & listen so kids will talk*. Scribner.

Falkenström, F., Granström, F., & Holmqvist, R. (2013). Therapeutic alliance predicts symptomatic improvement session by session. *Journal of Counseling Psychology, 60*(3), 317–328.

Feiler, B. (2013). *The secrets of happy families: Improve your mornings, tell your family history, fight smarter, go out and play, and much more*. Harper Collins.

Feller, C. P., & Cottone, R. R. (2012). The importance of empathy in the therapeutic alliance. *Journal of Humanistic Counseling, Education and Development, 42*(1), 53–61.

Fiese, B. H., Tomcho, T. J., Douglas, M., Josephs, K., Poltrock, S., & Baker, T. (2002). A review of 50 years of research on naturally occurring family routines and rituals: Cause for celebration? *Journal of Family Psychology, 16*, 381–390.

Fraiberg, S., Adelson, E., & Shapiro, V. (1975). Ghosts in the nursery: A psychoanalytic approach to the problems of impaired infant–mother relationships. *Journal of American Academy of Child Psychiatry, 14*(3), 387–421.

Frey, J., & Hall, A. (2021). *Motivational interviewing for mental health clinicians: A toolkit for skills enhancement*. PESI.

Frontline. (1994). *The trouble with Evan*. PBS. *www.pbs.org/wgbh/frontline/film/the-trouble-with-evan.*

Funderburk, B. W., & Eyberg, S. (2011). Parent–child interaction therapy. In J. C. Norcross, G. R. VandenBos, & D. K. Freedheim (Eds.), *History of psychotherapy: Continuity and change* (pp. 415–420). American Psychological Association.

Gartstein, M. A., Putnam, S. P., & Rothbart, M. K. (2012). Etiology of preschool behavior problems: Contributions of temperament attributes in early childhood. *Infant Mental Health Journal, 33*(2), 197–211.

Ginott, H. (2003). *Between parent and child: Revised and updated: The bestselling classic that revolutionized parent–child communication*. Three Rivers Press.

Goodman, S. H., & Brand, S. R. (2009). Infants of depressed mothers: Vulnerabilities, risk factors, and protective factors for the later development of psychopathology. In C. H. Zeanah, Jr. (Ed.), *Handbook of infant mental health* (3rd ed., pp. 153–170). Guilford Press.

Goodyear-Brown, P. (2021). *Parents as partners in child therapy: A clinician's guide*. Guilford Press.

Gopalan, G., Dean-Assael, K., Klingenstein, K., Chacko, A., & McKay, M. M. (2011). Caregiver depression and youth disruptive behavior difficulties. *Social Work in Mental Health, 9*(1), 56–70.

Gray, C. (2015). *The new social story book, revised and expanded 15th anniversary edition: Over 150 social stories that teach everyday social skills to children and adults with autism and their peers*. Future Horizons.

Greene, R. W. (1998). *The explosive child: A new approach for understanding and parenting easily frustrated, chronically inflexible children*. HarperCollins.

Greene, R. W. (2016). *Raising human beings: Creating a collaborative partnership with your child.* Scribner.

Greenspan, S. I., & Wieder, S. (2006). *Engaging autism: The floortime approach to helping children relate, communicate and think.* Perseus Books.

Gurley, J. R. (2011). Revised Children's Manifest Anxiety Scale: Second edition. In S. Goldstein & J. A. Naglieri (Eds.), *Encyclopedia of child behavior and development.* Springer.

Hatfield, E., Cacioppo, J. T., & Rapson, R. L. (1993). Emotion contagion. *Current Directions in Psychological Science, 2*(3), 96–99.

Hays, D. G., & Erford, B. T. (2017). *Developing multicultural counseling competence* (3rd ed.). Pearson.

Heath, C., & Heath, D. (2010). *Switch: How to change things when change is hard.* Broadway Books.

Hill, C. E., Spiegel, S. B., Hoffman, M., Kavlighan, Jr., D. M., & Gelso, C. J. (2017). Therapist expertise in psychotherapy revisited. *The Counseling Psychologist, 45*(1), 1–47.

Horvath, A. O. (2001). The alliance. *Psychotherapy: Theory, Research, Practice, Training, 38*(4), 365–372.

Houck, G. M., & LeCuyer-Maus, E. A. (2002). Maternal limit-setting patterns and toddler development of self-concept and social competence. *Issues in Comprehensive Pediatric Nursing, 25,* 21–41.

Huebner, D. (2005). *What to do when you worry too much.* Magination Press.

James, S. E., Herman, J. L., Rankin, S., Keisling, M., Mottet, L., & Anafi, M. (2016, December). *The report of the 2015 U.S. transgender survey.* National Center for Transgender Equality. Retrieved February 11, 2023, from *wwws://transequality.org/sites/default/files/docs/usts/USTS-Full-Report-Dec17.pdf.*

Kahanovitz, L., Sluss, P. M., & Russell, S. J. (2017). Type 1 diabetes—A clinical perspective. *Point of Care, 16*(1), 37–40.

Kandler, C., Riemann, R., & Angleitner, A. (2013). Patterns and sources of continuity and change of energetic and temporal aspects of temperament in adulthood: A longitudinal twin study of self- and peer reports. *Developmental Psychology, 49*(9), 1739–1753.

Karim, F., Oyewande, A. A., Abdalla, L. F., Chaudhry Ehsanullah, R., & Khan, S. (2020). Social media use and its connection to mental health: A systematic review. *Cureus, 12*(6), e8627.

Kawamichi, H., Yoshihara, K., Sasaki, A., & Sugawara, S. (2014). Perceiving active listening activates the reward system and improves the impression of relevant experiences. *Social Neuroscience, 10*(1), 1–11.

Kazdin, A. E. (2008). *The Kazdin method for parenting the defiant child: With no pills, no therapy, no contest of wills.* Houghton Mifflin.

Killgore, W. D. S. (2010). Effects of sleep deprivation on cognition. *Progress in Brain Research, 185,* 105–129.

Kinniburgh, K. (2014, November 7). *Treating complex childhood trauma: Targeting the building blocks of resilience.* ARC Training.

Klotz, L. (2021). *Subtract: The untapped science of less.* Flatiron Books.

Kohl, A., Rief, W., & Glombiewski, J. A. (2013). Acceptance, cognitive restructuring, and distraction as coping strategies for acute pain. *Journal of Pain, 3,* 305–315.

Kohn, A. (1993). *Punished by rewards: The trouble with gold stars, incentive plans, A's, praise, and other bribes.* Houghton Mifflin.

Kohn, A. (2005). *Unconditional parenting: Moving from rewards and punishments to love and reason.* Simon & Schuster.

Kohn, A. (2006). *The homework myth: Why our kids get too much of a bad thing.* Perseus Book Group.

Kopala-Sibley, D. C., Olino, T., Durbin, E., Dyson, M. W., & Klein, D. N. (2018). The stability of temperament from early childhood to early adolescence: A multi-method, multi-informant examination. *European Journal of Personality, 32*(2), 128–145.

Kornfield, J. (n.d.). *Parenting as practice.* Retrieved April 20, 2022, from *wwws://jackkornfield.com/parenting-practice.*

Lamborn, S. D., Mounts, N. S., Steinberg, L., & Dornbusch, S. M. (1991). Patterns of competence and adjustment among adolescents from authoritative, authoritarian, indulgent, and neglectful families. *Child Development, 62*(5), 1049–1065.

Landreth, G. L. (2002). Therapeutic limit setting in the play therapy relationship. *Professional Psychology: Research and Practice, 33*(6), 529–535.

Lavrič, M., & Naterer, A. (2020). The power of authoritative parenting: A cross-national study of effects of exposure to different parenting styles on life satisfaction. *Children and Youth Services Review, 116,* 105274.

Lieberman, A. F., Dimmler, M. H., & Ghosh Ippen, C. M. (2019). Child–parent psychotherapy: A trauma-informed treatment for young children and their caregivers. In C. H. Zeanah, Jr. (Ed.), *Handbook of infant mental health* (4th ed., pp. 485–499). Guilford Press.

Lieberman, A. F., Padrón E., Van Horn P., & Harris, W. W. (2005). Angels in the nursery: The intergenerational transmission of benevolent parental influences. *Infant Mental Health Journal, 26*(6), 504–520.

Lieberman, A. F., & Van Horn, P. (2011). *Psychotherapy with infants and young children: Repairing the effects of stress and trauma on early attachment.* Guilford Press.

Lieneman, C. C., Brabson, L. A., Highlander, A., Wallace, N. M., & McNeil, C. B. (2017). Parent–child interaction therapy: Current perspectives. *Psychology Research and Behavior Management, 10,* 239–256.

Linehan, M. (1993). *Cognitive-behavioral treatment of borderline personality disorder.* Guilford Press.

Linehan, M. (2014). *DBT skills training manual* (2nd ed.). Guilford Press.

Mabe, P. A., Turner, M. K., & Josephson, A. M. (2001). Parent management training. *Child and Adolescent Psychiatric Clinics of North America, 10*(3), 451–464.

Main, M., Kaplan, N., & Cassidy, J. (1985). Security in infancy, childhood, and adulthood: A move to the level of representation. *Monographs of the Society for Research in Child Development, 50*(1–2), 66–104.

March, J. S., & Benton, C. M. (2007). *Talking back to OCD: The program that helps kids and teens say "no way"—and parents say "way to go."* Guilford Press.

Marshall, M. (2010). *Parenting without stress: How to raise responsible kids while keeping a life of your own.* Piper Press.

Marshman, Z., Ahern, S. M., McEachen, R. R. C., Rogers, H. J., Gray-Burrows, K. A., & Day, P. F. (2016). Parents' experiences of toothbrushing with children: A qualitative study. *JDR Clinical and Translational Research, 1,* 122–130.

Mash, E. J., & Hunsley, J. (2007). Assessment of child and family disturbance: A developmental-systems approach. In E. J. Mash & R. A. Barkley (Eds.), *Assessment of childhood disorders* (4th ed., pp. 3–50). Guilford Press.

Maslow, A. H. (1943). A theory of human motivation. *Psychological Review, 50*(4), 370–396.

McElwain, A. (2019, June 24). Do our taste buds change with age: Now we know: Children's sense tends to be sharper as we lose buds as we get older. *Irish Times.* Retrieved from *www.irishtimes.com/life-and-style/food-and-drink/do-our-taste-buds-change-with-age-1.3922386#.*

McKenna, J. J., & McDade, T. (2005). Why babies should never sleep alone: A review of the co-sleeping controversy in relation to SIDS, bedsharing and breast feeding. *Paediatric Respiratory Reviews, 6*(2), 134–152.

McNeil, C. B., & Hembree-Kigin, T. L. (2010). *Parent–child interaction therapy* (2nd ed.). Springer.

Miller, A. L., Glinski, J., Woodberry, K. A., Mitchell, A. G., & Indik, J. (2002). Family therapy and dialectical behavior therapy with adolescents: Part I: Proposing a clinical synthesis. *American Journal of Psychotherapy, 56*(4), 568–584.

Miller, A. L., Rathus, J. H., & Linehan, M. M. (2007). *Dialectical behavior therapy with suicidal adolescents*. Guilford Press.

Miller, W. R., & Rollnick, S. (2013). *Motivational interviewing: Helping people to change* (3rd ed.). Guilford Press.

Mindell, J. A., & Williamson, A. A. (2018). Benefits of a bedtime routine in young children: Sleep, development, and beyond. *Sleep Medicine Reviews, 40*, 93–108.

Mogel, W. (2008). *The blessing of a skinned knee: Raising self-reliant children*. Simon & Schuster.

Montuclard, A. L., Park-Mroch, J., O'Shea, A. M. J., Wansinki, B., Irvin, J., & Laroche, H. H. (2017). College cafeteria signage increases water intake but water position on the soda dispenser encourages more soda consumption. *Journal of Nutrition Education and Behavior, 49*, 764–771.

Najdowski, A. C. (2017). *Flexible and focused: Teaching executive function skills to individuals with autism and attention disorders*. Elsevier.

Nassau, J., Buchanan, G. M., & High, P. C. (2009). Behavior management. In W. B. Carey, A. C. Crocker, W. L. Coleman, E. R. Elias, & H. M. Feldman (Eds.), *Developmental-behavioral pediatrics* (4th ed.). Elsevier.

National Association of Social Workers. (2017). NASW code of ethics. *www.socialworkers.org/About/Ethics/Code-of-Ethics/Code-of-Ethics-English*.

National Education Association. (2019, November 10). How much homework is too much? *NEA Today*. Retrieved from *www.nea.org/professional-excellence/student-engagement/tools-tips/how-much-homework-too-much*.

Newland, R. P., & Crnic, K. A. (2011). Mother–child affect and emotion socialization processes across the late preschool period: Predictions of emerging problem behavior. *Infant and Child Development, 20*, 371–388.

NSW (New South Wales) Government. (n.d.) *Your duties and rights as a parent*. Retrieved April 30, 2022, from *www.facs.nsw.gov.au/families/parenting/responsibility-and-rights/parent-duties*.

Owen, L., & Corfe, B. (2017). The role of diet and nutrition on mental health and well-being. *Proceedings of the Nutrition Society, 76*(4), 425–426.

Park, M., Tiwari, A., & Neumann, J. W. (2020). Emotional scaffolding in early childhood education. *Educational Studies, 46*(3), 570–589.

Paruthi, S., Brooks, L. J., D'Ambrosio, C., Hall, W. A., Kotagal, S., Lloyd, R. M., . . . Wise, M. S. (2016). Recommended amount of sleep for pediatric populations: A consensus statement of the American Academy of Sleep Medicine. *Journal of Clinical Sleep Medicine, 12*, 785–786.

Pascali, M., Matera, E., Craig, F., Torre, F., Giordano, P., Margari, F., . . . Margari, L. (2019). Cognitive, emotional, and behavioral profile in children and adolescents with chronic pain associated with rheumatic diseases: A case–control study. *Clinical Child Psychology and Psychiatry, 24*(3), 433–445.

Platania-Solazzo, A., Field, T. M., Blank, J., Seligman, F., Kuhn, C., Schanberg S., & Saab, P. (1992). Relaxation therapy reduces anxiety in child and adolescent psychiatric patients. *Acta Paedopsychiatrica, 55*(2), 115–120.

Posada, G., Jacobs, A., Richmond, M. K., Carbonell, O. A, Alzate, G., Bustamante, M. R., & Quiceno, J. (2002). Maternal caregiving and infant security in two cultures. *Developmental Psychology, 38*(1), 67–78.

Powell, B., Cooper, G., Hoffman, K., & Marvin, R. (2016). *The Circle of Security intervention: Enhancing attachment in early parent–child relationships*. Guilford Press.

Prochaska, J. O., & DiClemente, C. C. (1983). Stages and processes of self-change of smoking: Toward an integrative model of change. *Journal of Consulting and Clinical Psychology, 51*(3), 390–395.

Raby, K. L., Lawler, J. M., Shlafer, R. J., Hesemeyer, P. S., Collins, W. A., & Sroufe, L. A. (2015). The interpersonal antecedents of supportive parenting: A prospective, longitudinal study from infancy to adulthood. *Developmental Psychology, 51*(1), 115–123.

Rapee, R., Wignall, A., Spence, S. H., Cobham, V., & Lyneham, H. (2009). *Helping your anxious child: A step-by-step guide for parents.* New Harbinger.

Rodriguez-Ayllon, M., Cadenas-Sánchez, C., Estévez-López, F., Muñoz, N. E., Mora-Gonzalez, J., Migueles, J. H., . . . Esteban-Cornejo, I. (2019). Role of physical activity and sedentary behavior in the mental health of preschoolers, children and adolescents: A systematic review and meta-analysis. *Sports Medicine, 49,* 1383–1410.

Rushton, J. P. (1975). Generosity in children: Immediate and long-term effects of modeling, preaching, and moral judgment. *Journal of Personality and Social Psychology, 31,* 459–466.

Sameroff, A. (2009). The transactional model. In A. Sameroff (Ed.), *The transactional model of development: How children and contexts shape each other* (pp. 3–21). American Psychological Association.

Scharff, M., Mayseless, O., & Kivenson-Baron, I. (2004). Adolescents' attachment representations and developmental tasks in emerging adulthood. *Developmental Psychology, 40*(3), 430–444.

Scheeringa, M. S., & Zeanah, C. H. (2001). A relational perspective on PTSD in early childhood. *Journal of Traumatic Stress, 14*(4), 799–815.

Schmall, T. (2018, October 3). Parents get way less than an hour per day of "me time." *New York Post.*

Scott, H. K., Jain, A., & Cogburn, M. (Updated 2023, July 10). Behavior modification. In *StatPearls* [Internet]. StatPearls Publishing. Available at *www.ncbi.nlm.nih.gov/books/NBK459285.*

Sears, W., & Sears, M. (2001). *The attachment parenting book: A commonsense guide to understanding and nurturing your baby.* Little, Brown.

Sege, R. D., Siegel, B. S., Council on Child Abuse and Neglect, & Committee on Psychosocial Aspects of Child and Family Health. (2018). Effective discipline to raise healthy children. *Pediatrics, 142*(6), e20183112.

Sherif, M., Harvey, O. J., White, B. J., Hood, W. R., & Sherif, C. W. (1961). *Intergroup conflict and cooperation: The Robbers Cave experiment* (Vol. 10). University Book Exchange.

Shlafer, R. J., Raby, K. L., Lawler, J. M., Hesemeyer, P. S., & Roisman, G. I. (2015). Longitudinal associations between adult attachment states of mind and parenting quality. *Attachment & Human Development, 17*(1), 83–95.

Siegel, J. P. (2004). Identification as a focal point in couple therapy. *Psychoanalytic Inquiry, 24*(3), 406–419.

Skenazy, L. (2009). *Free range kids: Giving our children the freedom we had without going nuts with worry.* Jossey-Bass.

Slone, N. C., & Owen, J. (2015). Therapist alliance activity, therapist comfort, and systemic alliance on individual psychotherapy outcome. *Journal of Psychotherapy Integration, 25*(4), 275–288.

Smith, B. L. (2012). The case against spanking: Physical discipline is slowly declining as some studies reveal lasting harms for children. *APA Monitor, 43*(4), 60.

Somers, V. (2007). Schizophrenia: The impact of parental illness on children. *British Journal of Social Work, 37,* 1319–1334.

Sroufe, L. A., Egeland, B., Carlson, E. A., & Collins, W. A. (2005). *The development of the person: The Minnesota Study of Risk and Adaptation from Birth to Adulthood.* Guilford Press.

Sturge-Apple, M. L., Davies, P. T., & Cummings, E. M. (2006). Impact of hostility and withdrawal in intraparental conflict on parental emotional unavailability and children's adjustment difficulties. *Child Development, 77,* 1623–1641.

Sue, D. W., Sue, D., Neville, H. A., & Smith, L. (2019). *Counseling the culturally diverse: Theory and practice* (8th ed.) Wiley.

Taveras, E. M., Rifas-Shiman, S., Bub, K. L., Gillman, M. W., & Oken, E. (2017). Prospective study of insufficient sleep and neurobehavioral functioning among school-age children. *Behavioral Concerns and Mental Health, 17,* 625–632.

Toth, S. L., Maughan, A., Manly, J. T., Spagnola, M., & Cicchetti, D. (2002). The relative efficacy of two interventions in altering maltreated preschool children's representational models: Implications for attachment theory. *Development and Psychopathology, 14,* 877–908.

Tracey, T. J., Bludworth, J., & Glidden-Tracey, C. E. (2012). Are there parallel processes in psychotherapy supervision? An empirical examination. *Psychotherapy (Chicago), 49*(3), 330–343.

Trad, P. V. (1992). *The theory and practice of previewing.* Wiley.

Webster-Stratton, C., & Reid, M. J. (2010). Parents, teachers, and therapists using child-directed play therapy and coaching skills to promote children's social and emotional competence and build positive relationships. In C. E. Schaefer (Ed.), *Play therapy for preschool children* (pp. 245–273). American Psychological Association.

Weekly, T., Walker, N., Beck, J., Akers, S., & Weaver, M. (2018). A review of apps for calming, relaxation, and mindfulness interventions for pediatric palliative care patients. *Children, 5*(2), 16.

Weinstein, M. (2006). *The surprising power of family meals: How eating together makes us smarter, stronger, healthier, and happier.* Steerforth Press.

Werner, E. E., & Smith, R. S. (1992). *Overcoming the odds: High risk children from birth to adulthood.* Cornell University Press.

Whittingham, K., & Coyne, L. (2019). *Acceptance and commitment therapy: The clinician's guide for supporting parents.* Academic Press.

Winner, M. G. (2007). *Thinking about you, thinking about me: Teaching perspective taking and social thinking to persons with social cognitive learning challenges* (2nd ed.). Think Social.

Worrall, H., Schweizer, R., Marks, E., Yuan, L., Lloyd, C., & Ramjan, R. (2018). The effectiveness of support groups: A literature review. *Mental Health and Social Inclusion, 22*(2), 85–93.

Xie, J., Xie, C., & Yang, W. (2020). The effect of hunger on cognition and its mechanism. *Advances in Psychological Science, 28,* 141–149.

Yogman, M., Garner, A., Hutchinson, J., Hirsh-Pasek, K., & Michnick Golinkoff, R. (2018). The power of play: A pediatric role in enhancing development in young children. *Pediatrics, 142*(3).

Zisser, A., & Eyberg, S. M. (2010). Parent–child interaction therapy and the treatment of disruptive behavior disorders. In J. R. Weisz & A. E. Kazdin (Eds.), *Evidence-based psychotherapies for children and adolescents* (pp. 179–193). Guilford Press.

Index

Note. f after a page number indicates a figure.

S

T